PICTURE PERFECT WEIGHT LOSS

THE VISUAL GUIDE TO PERMANENT WEIGHT LOSS

Dr Howard M. Shapiro

RODALE

This edition first published in 2004 by
Rodale Ltd
7–10 Chandos Street
London W1G 9AD
www.rodale.co.uk

© 2004 Rodale Ltd
Adapted from the original edition first published in the United States in 2000 by Rodale, Inc
Text © 2000–2004 Dr Howard M. Shapiro
Original photographs © Kurt Wilson/Rodale Images and Lou Manna (see below)
New photography © Rodale Ltd

Printed and bound by Shenzhen Donnelley Bright Sun Printing Co., Ltd
1 3 5 7 9 8 6 4 2

A CIP record for this book is available from the British Library
ISBN 1-4050-3335-5

This paperback edition distributed to the book trade by Pan Macmillan Ltd

Produced for Rodale Books International by

studio cactus ©

Food styling by Annie Nichols
Book design by Sharon Rudd and Briony Chappell
Edited by Laura Seber

Cover photography by Jeremy Hopley (croissant and butter = 410 calories/fruit = 410 calories).
Interior photographs by Jeremy Hopley except: Kurt Wilson/Rodale Images: pages 17, 25, 29, 31
(chicken noodle soup; vegetable soup; baked apple), 35, 51, 69, 74 (smoked salmon), 76 (cheddar),
83, 86, 122, 123, 127, 129, 159. Lou Manna: pages 90, 91. Nigel James: pages 110, 118, 119.
Stockbyte: pages 8, 45, 133, 137, 161. PhotoDisc: pages 11, 32, 46, 138, 143, 145, 148, 149, 151, 157.
Studio Cactus: pages 13, 14, 31 (fruit yoghurt), 70, 72 (snack bar). Corbis: page 141.

www.drhowardshapiro.com

Notice
This book is intended as a reference volume only, not as a medical manual. The information given
here is designed to help you make informed decisions about your health. It is not intended as a
substitute for any treatment that may have been prescribed by your doctor. If you suspect that you
have a medical problem, we urge you to seek competent medical help.

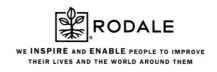

RODALE
WE INSPIRE AND ENABLE PEOPLE TO IMPROVE
THEIR LIVES AND THE WORLD AROUND THEM

To My Grandparents
Ida and Max Gallner
"They don't make them like that anymore."

To My Father
Charles Shapiro
May 23, 1915–September 14, 1999
Thank you for sharing the completion of this book.

To My Mother
Eleanor Gallner
November 30, 1920–August 12, 2002
Who encouraged me to realise my dreams.

CONTENTS

YES, IT'S OKAY TO EAT!

Fed up with diets? You're not alone. For nearly 20 years, I have specialised in weight control at my practice in mid-Manhattan. In addition to being the financial, shopping and theatre capital of the United States, New York City is also the diet capital.

Many of my patients are celebrities in the worlds of media, entertainment and fashion. You can imagine how important it is to look good if you're constantly in the limelight. For them, looking attractive and stylish is a job requirement. Of course they want to feel healthy and look great for personal reasons, too. But even more compelling than that are their professional reasons. This is something that has to happen for the sake of their careers.

Others are leaders in business and politics. To look powerful and in control, they have to appear healthy and fit. For them as well, losing weight is a very serious business.

I used to think New Yorkers were unique in their weight concerns. But of course they're not. Millions of people across the world want to lose weight. And they're searching for the best way to do it.

WHEN DIETS DON'T DO IT

I've met thousands of people who were fed up with diets. These are people who vowed 'Never again!' – and meant it. Many of the people who come through my door have have tried dozens of diets. Many are hardened and cynical survivors of yo-yo dieting, that infamous and health-sapping pattern of drastically losing weight while dieting only to put it on again as soon as the diet is over. And yet these hardened sceptics are still willing to visit a 'weight-loss doctor'.

Why? The fact is, these people come to me because they don't want the same kind of diets they've tried before. Indeed, they're ready to run from those kinds of diets. They want a weight-loss plan that doesn't leave them feeling deprived, hungry and unhappy. They're asking for some way to help them lose weight and keep it off while they continue with their busy, active lifestyles.

Even though weight loss is vital to the careers of many of my clients, it doesn't mean that it's easier for these people than it is for you and me. The only difference is that they can't afford to fail. To lose weight and keep it off, many of them are willing to pay thousands of pounds. They get personal counselling – my staff work with each person individually. But the secrets to their weight-loss successes, the reasons why they have succeeded and recommend me to others, are all in this book.

While you won't get personal coaching and counselling from this book, I can assure

You'll never have to count calories or grams of fat

you that you will be able to get many of the same weight-loss benefits from it. You'll feel better, you'll look better and you won't have to go through the heartbreaking cycle of losing weight only to put it back on again. Best of all, you won't have to stop eating.

Once you've developed Food Awareness Training using the techniques in this book, you don't have to think about all the food that 'thin people can eat'. You don't have to avoid restaurants or avoid dinner invitations.

After Food Awareness Training, weight loss becomes automatic because you react automatically. I know this takes some explaining, but first, I'd like to give you some understanding of what lies behind this remarkable programme.

LOOK – NO BAD FOODS!

Soon after I opened my weight-loss clinic, I made a discovery that has affected everything I've done since. I discovered a simple truth: no single weight-loss programme can work for everyone.

> I don't tell my patients what they should or shouldn't eat

Of course, we'd all like an easy solution to the problem of losing weight. Many people have spent a lot of time and money trying to work out how. Some have even put their health at risk in search of the quick, magic fix. Early in my practice, I began to encounter people who had been on many types of strange diets. Some ate extremely large or small quantities of food. Others tried bizarre combinations. Still others pursued programmes that included pills and injections.

But I didn't have a 'Dr Shapiro Diet', and I still don't. When people leave my office, they don't carry handouts listing the foods that they should and shouldn't eat at various times of the day. I never ask patients to alter their usual routines, and that's probably a good thing, since most of them can't. As you've probably discovered yourself, you can't leave your job or change your family or cancel holidays just because you need to lose weight. Weight loss – or maintenance – needs to be something that happens while you're still getting on with your life.

I don't tell my patients what to eat. Instead, I talk about the choices that they can make. I ask them to subscribe to a few principles that, I believe, are the essential components of successful weight loss:

■ **ANY REASON FOR EATING IS OKAY:** For years, people on diets were told: 'Eat only when you're hungry.' Research has shown, however, that there's no clear line between the physiological and the emotional reasons for eating. So asking someone to decide whether they have a real, physical need for food is asking for the impossible. If you're deprived of food for any reason, you're likely to have an increased need to eat. And the more you deny that need, the more food-obsessed you can become. So what should you do if you crave food?

I think you should go right ahead and have some. Sometimes, that means you'll eat when you're not physically hungry, but that's okay. You really do want to eat. Just eat the healthiest and lowest-calorie foods that you find satisfying.

■ **THERE ARE NO BAD FOODS:** Sweets are okay. Desserts are okay. You're not 'cheating' if you eat those foods, but you are making choices. Yes, there are times when only the high-fat, high-calorie food will do. But there are also many alternatives.

■ **THERE ARE NO 'CORRECT' PORTIONS:** Hunger varies from person to person. The need for food goes up and down. Even if you eat a whole tub of sorbet or a dozen boiled sweets, the diet isn't a failure. Sure, you've eaten a lot because you were hungry, for whatever reason, but you haven't blown your weight-loss plan. You're still in the driver's seat. You're not out of control. Don't worry about 'getting back on track' because you're never off track.

■ **YOU'RE NEVER ON A DIET:** Instead of dieting, you're participating in an on-going process of learning to make satisfying food choices. On a typical deprivation diet, people often eat ravenously as soon as the diet is over. With Food Awareness Training, you never feel this kind of deprivation. You'll adopt new eating habits that you'll find completely comfortable.

A VIEW OF YOUR OPTIONS

Food Awareness Training begins when you see your food choices. When patients come to my office, the nutritionist sets up actual food or meals for visual demonstrations.

These demonstrations help people take the first step towards developing a new

> **One look is all it takes to help you make your choices**

relationship with food. That's the first lesson in Food Awareness Training. It really doesn't take much to make us aware of what we're eating, but sometimes you simply have to see it to believe it.

With Food Awareness Training, you don't have to count calories. Instead, simply think of the pictures in this book. Turn now to the pictures on pages 70–71. Look how much you can eat instead of that croissant. Even if you were starving, it's unlikely that you could eat all the food to the right of the equals sign.

I'm not saying that you can't eat the croissant. Of course you can. But you can also see what your options are. Very clearly.

If you're reading this book, you have probably dieted before and may consider yourself fairly knowledgeable about weight loss. So you probably know the cold, hard mathematical facts about food, fat and calories. Rationally, logically, you could get out a calorie guide and a calculator and work out how many calories you're getting from each food. But who has time for all that?

The reason why this food demonstration works so effectively is that the images appeal to a different part of your brain. Instead of calculating your choices, you can see your choices. Research shows that when visual

YOUR LIFESTYLE

Many of my patients travel and entertain. They have business engagements where contacts are made and deals are done over drinks, lunch or dinner. Can they give up these appointments? Of course not. And neither can you if business meals are a necessary part of your professional life. What you can do, however, is take control of these situations. You can continue your normal activities as you work towards losing weight. Once you've lost weight, you can maintain that loss by continuing to make the best choices.

Even if you're not a power luncher, other challenges may be built into your lifestyle. Take breakfast, for example: some people just grab something and go. I won't try to change that pattern. If you're used to grabbing breakfast on the run, so be it. What you can do is choose what you eat for that 'quickie' breakfast. Or you may be someone who's home all day, with the kitchen near at hand. You can't change the circumstances, but there are things you can do to ensure that you're making the right choices without depriving yourself.

images are stored in your memory, you retain them longer. And they have much greater impact on your behaviour, so you can make the right food choices instinctively.

As a result of looking at the pictures in this book and reading the accompanying explanations, better food choices will become a matter of routine. You'll experience the pleasure that comes not only from having eaten, but also from having eaten amply, wisely and well.

NO QUICK-FIX TRAPS

For anyone who starts to put on weight, a gimmick diet might appear to offer a quick fix. My advice: stay away from those diets. You need practical, easy-to-understand information to make some healthy and easy adjustments to the way you choose food.

With my programme, you can continue to eat real food, and you don't have to follow a set routine of eating a certain amount at a particular time. Also, you don't have to deal with control and deprivation. While you're eating healthier food – for some people, the best food they've ever had in their lives – you'll also be controlling your weight, as long as you have Food Awareness Training to guide the hand that feeds you.

If you have gone on diets many times during your life, you'll be relieved to discover that Food Awareness doesn't involve unusual regimes and extremes of deprivation. I know how extraordinary those programmes can be, having met people who have tried everything from injections to elaborate rituals that involve weighing each portion of food. Food Awareness Training will teach you how to make food choices that can apply for a lifetime.

With this plan, you have the very best chance of losing weight and keeping it off – without ever feeling deprived. Most importantly, you won't have to go through the heartbreaking cycle of losing and gaining weight again. You will never have to see a dietician or join a programme. Why? Because you will be dealing with food in a totally different way than you ever have before.

MAKING THE RIGHT CHOICES

If you're particularly concerned about fitness and nutrition, Food Awareness Training will help guide you through the maze of information and apparent contradictions that relate to reduced-fat or low-calorie foods and drinks. Which of these foods really do make sense? With Food Awareness Training, you'll find out which of the supposed diet foods are nutritional booby traps and learn to make other choices automatically. You'll also discover some of the nutritional superstars that can help you maintain a well-balanced, healthy diet even if you're trying to maintain or lose weight.

> ## You won't feel hungry because you'll be eating a lot

If you're a teenager or college student, you may already think a lot about being overweight. But even if you know that certain foods should be avoided, you may not always find it convenient to sit down to regular meals. Also, you may not be sure which foods are good choices for meals or snacking. With Food Awareness Training, you can pick up knowledge of your food choices with minimum effort.

This book presents the information you need to make your choices in a memorable and easy-to-understand way. You can start to develop automatic eating habits that will help you for the rest of your life.

SEEING IS BELIEVING

Does it seem to you that everywhere you go, people are talking about their diets?

It's true. In millions of homes each day, clock radios go off and people get out of bed, go into the bathroom, look in the mirror and think about a diet. However, only a tiny proportion of these people are actually dieting at any given time.

What happens to all the other promises? They're broken as soon as the man in the too-tight shirt reaches for that piece of Danish pastry in the bustle of the morning meeting. For the mum who's at home with the kids, the diet promise ends as soon as she takes a few more nibbles of the kids' snack foods because she needs energy. For the person who has been chained to a desk all day, trying hard not to think about food, the diet promise comes to a crashing end with a late-night bowl of ice cream.

People who are overweight are more likely to need surgery

Everyone knows that being overweight isn't good for you. The insurance companies certainly know it: to determine risk groups, they have gathered masses of statistics about what happens to people who are overweight. They've realised that if you're overweight, you're more prone to diseases such as heart disease and diabetes, or from suffering from a stroke or high blood pressure. People who are overweight are more likely to need surgery, and once they've had the surgery, they're more likely to develop complications. Being overweight even affects your buying power:

those who weigh more are likely to earn less money, especially if they're executives.

ENOUGH INCENTIVES?

Better health and more prosperity are fine motivators. But even with these incentives, the thought of going on a diet is difficult to contemplate.

Food Awareness Training is flexible, not boring

A diet is rigid. A diet is boring. A diet means giving up all the foods you like. A diet means changing your lifestyle. A diet means feeling hungry. And many people have discovered something else that's incredibly discouraging about diets: once they're over, you usually begin to put the weight back on.

Before you start to take the first steps towards Food Awareness Training, I want you to get rid of all those thoughts about dieting. This is not like any other diet you may have known. You do not have to give up the food you love or change your lifestyle. You will never feel hungry. You will change your entire relationship with food so you need never be on the same up-and-down weight cycle again.

This is not a 'diet book' in any conventional sense. Start with the fact that it is not just for dieters. You won't have to rely on prescriptions, diet gurus, or prepared meals. While this book will help anyone who is trying to lose weight, either through an individual or group programme or with the help of a doctor, it is also meant to help people who are trying to maintain weight, eat in a healthier way or make better choices for their children.

WILL IT WORK FOR ME?

Of course, the way you approach Food Awareness Training is likely to be influenced by experiences that you've had with diet or weight-loss programmes in the past. Fortunately, the programme has worked both for those who have never tried diets and for those who have been through numerous plans and programmes that were designed to help them lose weight.

Food Awareness Training is just as effective for men as it is for women, and just as effective for young people as it is for those who are middle-aged or older.

If you've never been concerned with weight loss, but you are now, Food Awareness Training can help you make food choices that ensure you'll never have to go on a drastic weight-loss programme. In fact, many people who come to see me are experiencing a weight problem for the first time.

Among the first-timers are women who notice small to moderate weight gain with the onset of menopause. The extra weight isn't a problem, and they want to make sure it doesn't become one. They feel like there are certain things that they can do now to lose some weight and avoid a lot of weight gain in the future. And they're right.

My programme works for a wide range of people

Some men meet their first challenge with weight gain just as they're reaching middle age. That's to be expected. Metabolisms change as we get older, and the food that we consume doesn't get burned up as quickly. Even if our eating habits don't change, it's easy to put on a few pounds – and much harder to take them off. In fact, by the time

THE KEY TO WEIGHT LOSS

When I was beginning my practice, I prescribed many different approaches to losing weight that were tailored to individual needs. I discovered that calorie reduction is the key.

On a long-term basis, there is only one safe, effective, foolproof way to get yourself down to a lower weight and keep off the extra pounds. That is to eat a healthy, reduced-calorie diet and get enough exercise.

I also found that most people don't enjoy counting calories. First-time dieters quickly discover that it's a time-consuming and complicated chore. Calorie counting almost always goes hand in hand with the feeling of being deprived that spells doom to a diet. That realisation led to the next step in developing my programme: demonstrations that help you remember which choices to make.

The really good news is that eating fewer calories does not necessarily mean eating less food. And it definitely doesn't mean that you have to walk around in a constant state of deprivation. After all, a feeling of deprivation is the surest way to make your weight-loss plan fail. Instead, you may be eating even more food. You will certainly feel satisfied.

you're a mature adult, you need 100 fewer daily calories than you needed when you were growing up.

Some people who have never had weight problems in the past find that a new medication can have side effects. For example, people often gain weight if they start taking drugs that contain steroids. And some people gain weight when they have hormone therapy or take psychotropic medications such as antidepressants.

Other factors that can cause weight gain? Maybe you've put on a few pounds because you've started travelling for business a lot more than you used to. Or perhaps you have young children who tie you to the home front and kitchen much more than in the past. Working odd shifts, changing jobs or moving house can also initiate weight gain.

If you have gone on diets before, you'll be relieved to discover that Food Awareness doesn't involve unusual regimes and extremes of deprivation. With this plan, you have the best chance of losing weight and keeping it off – without ever feeling deprived.

SAME TASTE, FEWER CALORIES

Unfortunately, most veteran dieters expect the acceptable foods to be something like lettuce leaves and celery stalks. But if you flick through this book, you'll see many pictures of foods like bread and pizza, chunky soup, scallops with black bean sauce, curries and casseroles, snacks and sundaes. We're suggesting foods that you may decide to eat instead of high-calorie foods while getting the same satisfying taste.

Let's run a quick test right now. Do you like chocolate ice cream? Okay, you can have the richest chocolate ice cream available – for about 1000 calories for half a litre. Or you can have chocolate frozen yogurt or

sorbet, which have around 600 calories for half a litre. You will have satisfied your hunger for a lot fewer calories.

Look at the pictures on the following pages: these will show you what I'm talking about. And I guarantee, with these pictures firmly planted in the part of your brain that records visual images, you'll think very differently about the choices that you're making when you have a craving.

We see so much information about fat and calories that this information may seem pretty basic to most of us. But it's not always easy to judge the facts given to you. For instance, if you read a product label, you may register the fact that a food is 'high in fat' or 'low in fat', but you're less likely to pay attention to how this relates to serving size.

Just for fun, you might want to test some of the assumptions you have about different types of food. The food quiz opposite will help you do that. After you've tried it, check your answers on page 14.

A MALE MESSAGE, TOO

Several years ago, most of the men who came to see me were concerned about a health problem associated with weight. Some had heart problems, and their doctors had told them that they absolutely had to lose weight to help prevent future heart attacks. Others felt threatened by what they had found out about their family histories, which suggested that they might be in line for future health problems, such as hardening of the arteries, diabetes or other weight-related problems. Again, their doctors' warnings gave them an urgent nudge towards my office.

These days, more men are concerned with appearance. Yes, health concerns are still the dominant issues, but I am seeing many more men than I used to, and they have other issues.

Are you ready to face the challenge? It's quite easy, actually. Just look at the pairs of 'food comparisons' in the pictures below and guess which food in each pair is lower in calories. The calories are based on the amount of food you see in the photographs.

Just from this short quiz, you'll get a better idea about which choices you're making the next time you see these foods. Even if you get 100 per cent correct on the quiz, the images will remind you of things that you already know about these foods. You'll discover even more, and expand your choices, as you continue reading this book.

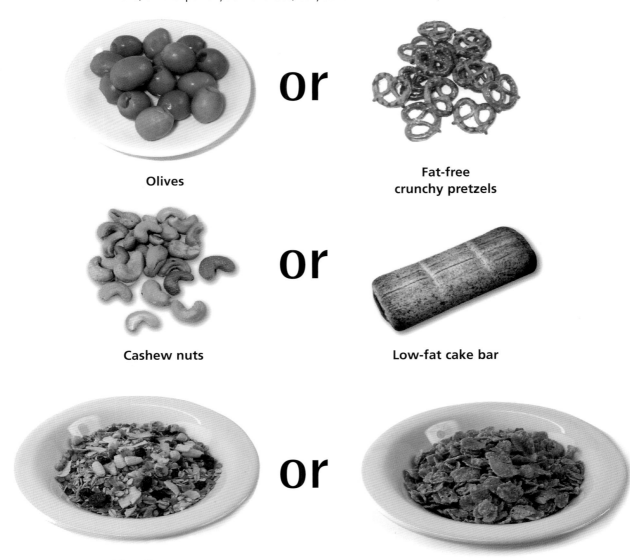

Olives

or

Fat-free crunchy pretzels

Cashew nuts

or

Low-fat cake bar

Muesli

or

Frosted flakes

ANSWERS TO QUIZ

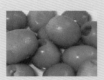
50g assorted olives = 80 calories

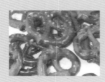
25g crunchy pretzels = 100 calories

Did you assume that the olives had the higher calorie count?

True, the pretzels look bare, dry and plain. Naturally, we're likely to assume that they must be low in calories. By contrast, we tend to think of olives as 'fattening' foods, and their lush appearance and rich taste only add to that image. It's accurate to say that olives contain fat, but many people don't realise they have the 'good' kind of fat – heart-healthy monounsaturated fat, not the saturated kind that raises artery-clogging cholesterol. As for calories, this dish of olives has only 80 calories – versus 100 calories for the bare, dry, plain, fat-free pretzels.

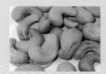
25g cashew nuts = 150 calories

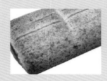
a low-fat cake bar = 150 calories

Low-fat cake bar versus cashew nuts? Seems like an easy choice, doesn't it?

It's hard to believe – but absolutely true – that this puny diet bar, the least cake-like cake around, has as many calories as a handful of cashew nuts, notorious for their fat content. And if this weren't enough, the cake bar is virtually nutrition-free, while the fats in the nuts are the essential fatty acids our bodies need.

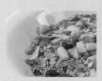
bowl of muesli (165g) = 650 calories

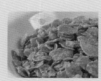
bowl of frosted flakes (42g) = 160 calories

At first glance, you probably thought this question was a dead giveaway: what could be higher in calories than a cereal that has been sweetened like crazy – frosted with sugar! – to make it more palatable to children? Against a healthy, grown-up offering like muesli, the kids' cereal, frosted flakes, probably seems like a non-contender.

In this case, however, the kids' 'junk' food is the better calorie bargain: 200 calories versus 250 calories for an equivalent portion of muesli. The fact is that almost all cereals have about 300 to 400 calories per 100g. The denser the cereal, the higher the calorie content per bowl. Muesli is a particularly dense cereal. It may be full of healthy fruit – but if you add some extra fruit to your frosted flakes you'll get the same benefits.

To convert calories to kilojoules, see page 166.

HELP FROM THE DEMOS

The food demonstrations not only help you choose wisely but also help you interpret nutritional information correctly. Here, too, the advice of dieticians and nutritionists is extremely valuable. We find, for example, that many people have mistaken beliefs about what they should and should not eat.

Take the term 'fat-free'. Thinking that fats should be avoided, many people believe that they can lose weight if they simply eliminate butter and oil from their diets.

What happens if you eat fat-free cakes and biscuits instead of the conventional fat-filled kind? What if you eat bagels instead of croissants? What if you have jelly beans instead of a chocolate bar, or pasta instead of a burger? Isn't weight loss guaranteed for people who adopt these fat-cutting strategies?

If that's what you've heard, and you've moved over to a low-fat or fat-free diet, then you may wonder why the bathroom scales aren't moving downwards. Where's the flaw in the low-fat reasoning?

Here's the problem: a fat-free cake, as advertised, is probably free of fat, but it is high in refined carbohydrates. Carbohydrate calories are very real calories. Like fat calories, they can either turn into energy when you exercise, or they can go to the fat

Carbohydrates can easily turn into body fat

cells in your body, where they're stored away. That's why food products that are advertised as 'fat-free' do not by themselves help you get thin.

When I speak to people who have had lifelong struggles with weight control, I tell them that the programme they will begin is not a short-term effort but the beginning of a journey during which their relationship with food will change. Even

You can eat a wide variety of foods that you really enjoy

very experienced dieters are surprised to discover that they don't have to stick with the foods that they thought were 'good' for them – foods they might not even like. Nothing I can say, however, drives home these points as powerfully as the food demonstrations.

THE LOOK OF KNOWLEDGE

One thing is certain once you've taken the quiz on the previous page: once you've seen the answers, you're unlikely to forget them. Seeing the actual food – and understanding how many calories are in that food – is a far more powerful message than reading a list of words and numbers.

These demonstrations – like the rest in this book – are likely to challenge many of your assumptions. Looking at their choices, people often say, 'That can't be true! How can one tiny low-fat snack bar have as many calories as all that fruit?'

But there's no trick to any of these demonstrations. Each one has been carefully checked, using all the information that we have about calorie counts, nutritional values and serving sizes, to make sure that the portions and amounts are accurate.

Since you're always making choices about what foods you eat and don't eat, I want to make sure that what you see is what you get – no optical illusions.

THE COSTS OF BEING OVERWEIGHT

In the past, the overwhelming majority of people who came to see me about weight control were women. Their number one concern was appearance. Many women just didn't like how they looked in jeans or bathing suits, and they wanted to change that. Few men seemed to share the same concerns. But that's starting to change. I am seeing a lot more men in my office, and appearance is often their number one reason for coming to see me.

Why are more men visiting me than before? Well, for one thing, there's been a change in our society, and men are no longer embarrassed to admit that they care about how they look. I see a lot more men working out, going to spas, colouring their hair, having cosmetic surgery – and coming to me to deal with their bodies.

The appearance factor is more than skin deep. Some top executives, for instance, now make room in their crowded diaries to visit my office to deal with their weight. Many male professionals have learnt – sometimes the hard way – that no one has a lifetime guarantee of employment. It is not unusual

People who are trim are perceived as being disciplined

for a Director or even a Chief Executive to be made redundant. If you are in the position of having to present yourself as a job candidate in competition with young people in good shape, you want to look as youthful, fit and healthy as possible. Fair or not, in many competitive business environments, being overweight is often seen as having a lack of willpower.

I've seen many men and women who were extremely talented, well-paid and promotable. But they understood that they could go even further in their careers if they were more 'presentable'. Many of my patients – both men and women – tell me that once they lost weight, they were suddenly treated differently at work.

Having been less sensitive about weight, some men have been slower to understand the professional and economic cost of being overweight. When they come to the door of my office, however, they're prepared to make some weight-loss choices that they feel will keep their options open.

As you begin using the information here, you may be facing similar issues in your professional life.

YOUR LIFESTYLE

You may not be a high-powered executive, but for every individual, there are huge benefits both to your health and to your self-esteem if you are not overweight. But whatever your lifestyle, there will be challenges where food is concerned.

I understand that you can't change your lifestyle just because you've decided to lose weight. Your lifestyle depends on such a wide range of factors – family, location, profession – that you need food choices that fit your lifestyle, rather than the other way around. That's why I do food demonstrations with so many different kinds of foods – not just things that you'll find in the cupboard or refrigerator but also with fast foods, street-vendor foods, takeaway and restaurant foods and common snacks.

The idea is to help you *see* your choices, no matter what circumstances you're in. The right solution is the one that helps you eat healthily, lose weight and not feel deprived.

MEET YOUR CHALLENGES

Over the course of my career, having interviewed thousands of people who are concerned with weight loss, I have discovered that each individual faces different challenges. However, many are in similar situations in terms of their lifestyles and schedules. Here are the four lifestyle situations that seem to pose the most problems.

TIED TO A DESK

Let's face it: many people who spend a lot of time in the office have fairly sedentary lifestyles. Lunch may be from a vending machine, the office cafeteria, or the local sandwich shop. Snacks are no further away than the desk drawer. If you're in this situation, you may find that you have a low-energy period in the late afternoon that you remedy with a 'sugar fix'. And, pressured by family demands or other obligations, you may be tempted to pick up convenience foods for breakfast or dinner.

WINED AND DINED

Executives who spend a lot of time doing business in social situations are likely to eat well but rarely on the same schedule from day to day. They may start their days with a 'power breakfast', hold a meeting at lunchtime and go to a social event for dinner. If your lifestyle is like this, you're probably travelling a great deal, often grabbing a bite to eat while you're on the road, in an airport, on a plane or in an hotel.

EATING ON THE RUN

If you have little time to eat, you may eat practically all your meals on the run. You get breakfast from a bakery or coffee shop. Lunch may be fast food. Dinner ends up being a takeaway. It's not uncommon to skip a meal, then eat as much as necessary to fill yourself up.

Young, single students are typical on-the-run eaters, but this pattern applies to anyone too busy to cook. Often, this eating style is driven by necessity and, in some professions, nearly everyone eats this way. Police officers, for instance, rarely have time for sit-down meals, except when they're off duty.

HOME WITH THE FAMILY

Stay-at-home mums and dads often have big snacking problems. When children leave food on their plates, parents hate to see it go to waste. So they take a bite here and there, and it all adds up. Also, in many families with children, it's likely there will be more junk food around. Crisps and biscuits find their way in, and it's all too easy to grab a handful while you're taking care of the family.

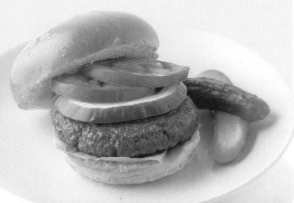

WHY YOU GAIN WEIGHT

As your own tastebuds will tell you again and again, food is not a villain. Most of us love it. And that's a good thing because we need food for growth and repair of tissues.

We need nutritional power to meet our energy needs

It's not the food itself but the storage process that makes us unhappy. If we eat more than we need for immediate use, our bodies put it into cosy, comfortable storage cells. Where are those cells located? You already know the answer. Most of the plump fat cells are located in the trouble spots that we know about – stomachs, hips, thighs, buttocks – as well as other areas that have fat-holding cells.

People who tend to be overweight have bodies that scientists would describe as efficient. Although efficiency might sound like a good thing, in the modern world it's a liability. If your body uses food efficiently, you get the energy you need immediately, and then store the excess.

Some people are lucky. Their bodies, almost mysteriously, don't store much of the food they eat. You know who I'm talking about – those few people who seem to be able to eat anything and still stay thin.

For the vast majority of us, however, the fat that we store just keeps hanging around. If only there were some way to reset the controls on our bodies. If we could do that, maybe we could turn the storage function from high to low.

Of course, as you know, scientists have not quite worked out a way to do this. Until they do, some people will be more likely to gain weight than others. The reasons have to do with body chemistry.

On the other hand, that doesn't mean your body is going to fight you all the way. Many people can maintain a significant degree of weight loss, but that's easiest to do when you don't feel deprived.

THE STRESS CONNECTION

Do you eat more or more erratically when you're feeling a lot of stress? For so many people, food is a stress reliever. And from what I have seen, people these days are under a lot more stress than they were in the past.

More women are juggling jobs and families. Men and women are spending longer hours at work. Many people hold down two jobs to maintain the high standard of living to which they aspire. And in many two-career families, time is at a premium.

Many people with careers also have to take on a large share of household responsibilities. After they get home, they have to look after home maintenance, cleaning, cooking, and child care. For so many of us, these are the stresses of everyday life that really add up.

Late-night snacking is not necessarily bad

The result? For many of us, food is a comfort and a reward. Only after the working day is over and the domestic duties are taken care of, can we sit back and relax. And that's when we reach for snack foods.

So what can we do? In my view, if this is the only time of day when you can get a break, why not enjoy it? But there are a number of satisfying and delicious snacks lower in calories than the ones you might normally reach for.

'GOOD' HUNGER

For many years, we were fed the myth that there was a difference between genuine hunger and mere appetite. Hunger was supposed to be a good, or normal, sensation that came after prolonged periods without food.

For years, we believed the myth that you could actually tell the difference between appetite and hunger. Experts said that if you hadn't eaten food for hours and were genuinely hungry, you would know it. Dizziness, weakness or acid stomach are the symptoms of real hunger.

Appetite, they claimed, was something different. Appetite was the result of out-of-control impulse. Your appetite, not hunger, made you head for the biscuit tin despite the fact that you had just finished dinner. If you polished off a whole bowl of peanuts while chatting with your friend at the bar, that was the fault of your appetite again.

By this reasoning, the hunger-versus-appetite dichotomy was black and white. If you were legitimately hungry, that was okay. But if your appetite was making you eat, well, that was deemed less acceptable, even shameful.

Appetite, we were told, was an emotional response rather than a biological one. Appetite led you to eat out of boredom or frustration or anger. Eating for emotional reasons sounds like a wrong reason to eat.

But as scientists have begun to unlock the secrets of weight gain and weight loss, they have learnt that people's reasons for eating can't be labelled in such neat and precise ways. The difference between hunger and appetite is hazy. Researchers have discovered that there are several hormones and neurochemicals in the body that have a profound effect on your life.

LISTEN TO YOUR CHEMICALS

There are at least six body chemicals that affect your weight. Their names are strange, and there's no reason to memorise them. But as weight-loss research continues, it's likely that you'll see these chemicals mentioned again and again. They are cholecystokinin, cortisol, dopamine, leptin, neuropeptide Y and serotonin.

At the moment, there are no adequate explanations about how each of these chemicals affects your weight. What researchers do know, however, is that these substances relay messages to your fat cells, blood, brain and intestines. They play a role in regulating body weight, appetite, eating behaviours and even the way you think about food.

The urge to eat is a need that must be filled

This is not to say that we are automatons programmed by chemicals. Our eating is also affected by other factors, from psyche to circumstances. Since the whole issue of eating is so complex, no researcher can tell you with absolute certainty why someone can resist the temptation of the bread basket one day but lust helplessly after chocolate cake the next day.

While it's nearly impossible to know the reasons why you need to eat a particular food at a particular time, it's very important to be in touch with that desire. You can't understand all the ways in which chemicals work, but you must listen when they talk to you. Most dieters have not learnt to do this. If we don't respond to our urges, the need-to-eat feelings will get the upper hand. As a result of trying not to respond to the need to eat, there's a good chance that you won't be able to lose weight or maintain weight loss.

BEYOND GOOD AND BAD

Most dieters have built-in defences. A statement as simple as 'I'm hungry!' is unacceptable to them. Before acknowledging something that simple, dieters are already worrying about how that hungry feeling may lead them into going astray, going out of control, or messing up. People who have been on diets tell me that they constantly feel either good or bad, in control or out of control.

But you can't repress a feeling that says, quite simply, 'I want to eat that'. You might try to keep that chemically driven impulse in check, but it's bound to get the upper hand.

Overweight individuals typically have so much anxiety about the urge to eat that their minds operate defensively. They don't even allow the hunger to come to consciousness. They find all kinds of rationalisations. For example, a person comes home from the supermarket with a cake, with the intention of serving it to friends. But lying just below the surface is the real reason for the purchase, which is simply her desire to eat cake.

What I'm telling you is something that you may have always suspected if you've struggled repeatedly with your weight – that the struggle is not being caused by a deficit in willpower. By identifying the chemicals that play a role in your hunger, we're beginning to get to the real causes. Soon, we should have the information that proves your suspicions are correct: gaining and losing weight are not matters of self-control, determination or other intangible factors.

Weight gain is not caused by lack of determination

In the meantime, that doesn't mean that your only choice is to throw up your hands and say, 'Well, it's fate. I was born to be overweight.' That is definitely not the case. You can reshape (literally) your destiny – or at least you can achieve the more modest goal of just shedding a few pounds.

DEPRIVATION DOESN'T WORK

To lose weight successfully, you either have to decrease your calorie intake or increase the number of calories expended through exercise – preferably both. To lose weight successfully and keep it off, you have to accomplish calorie reduction without feeling deprived. This is a key concept, and it is at the heart of my programme. Feeling deprived comes around and kicks you in the rear end – right in the direction of the nearest ice cream or cream cake.

I have been working with dieters for many years, and I know that they do not have a problem with willpower. Quite the reverse. People who can cling to a rigid diet, despite everything else that's going on in their lives, have unusual discipline. Some have managed to stick with extremely rigorous programmes for an amazingly long time

IN COMMAND OF APPETITE

Deep in the command centre of your brain, a protein with a funny name may play a role in telling you whether you're feeling full. The newly discovered protein, GLP-1, is made in a part of the brain called the hypothalamus. When you eat, GLP-1 tells the intestines and pancreas to slow down digestion. In animal studies, rats injected with GLP-1 showed signs that they were full before they finished their normal rations of food. When an inhibitor of GLP-1 was injected, the rats ate more than usual and grew fatter. More research is needed, however, before scientists can establish the role of GLP-1 in humans.

to reach their target weight. I have had people who stayed on a liquid protein fast without a morsel of real food for as long as 4 months. Don't tell me this demonstrates a lack of willpower!

I have also seen, however, many people who have worked unbelievably hard to reach a certain weight-loss goal, only to put all the weight back on. The feelings of deprivation were just too much for them, and once they had reached the numbers on the scale that they longed for, they resumed their old eating patterns. Yet, all the time they were dieting, they were not aware of feeling deprived.

People who are attempting to lose weight typically do not report feelings of deprivation; they bury them instead. They say that they had a bad week or that they ate because they weren't focused. They will say things like, 'I had plenty. I didn't need to eat the brownie'; 'I wasn't hungry' or 'I don't know why I did it'.

If those phrases sound familiar, I can assure you that people who are deprived of food do need to eat. If you eat, it's because you're hungry.

WHAT DIETS CAN DO TO YOU

Dieters don't eat unconsciously. They don't have blackouts. They know when they're eating the whole packet of biscuits. What they've blocked is the feeling of hunger. They tried to protect themselves from those urges.

A woman once came into my office reporting that she'd had a terrible week. She went to a birthday party that featured a lavish buffet. Smelling the food, she was tempted, but what really called out to her was a piece of cheesecake. She resisted it because she thought it was bad.

Instead of having the cheesecake, she had a cupcake that she thought was a little less

bad. The cupcake didn't satisfy her, so she had another cupcake. After that, she just continued eating, having far more food than she was comfortable with. She ate so quickly, and with such feelings of guilt, that she didn't enjoy any of it.

Work with your urges, or the inevitable result is a binge

What was the alternative? My message to her was that giving in to her urge and eating the cheesecake would not have been a problem. Where she had a problem was with her attitude. Instead of saying, 'This cheesecake looks good to me,' she said to herself, 'How can I avoid this cheesecake?'

HAVING YOUR CAKE AND YOUR WAISTLINE, TOO

It is a mistake to put eating on hold, to think that you can turn off your desire to eat as if you were turning off a switch. You will have the urge to eat cake or whatever else tempts you from time to time. That urge is not an evil thing. You don't have to view eating a piece of cake, or whatever you desire, as an unfortunate or disastrous lapse of self-control.

Get comfortable with your urges. It's okay to eat, as long as you do it mindfully. To lose weight successfully, you have to work out a way to have that occasional piece of cake and still feel like you're in the driver's seat. Work out a way to recognise the foods that you enjoy and then put them into your eating plan. Yes, that includes food like cakes and biscuits.

Try to become aware of the times when you experience the feeling of wanting to eat. It's perfectly okay to want food because you feel bored, frustrated or anxious. Remember: there is no wrong reason to eat.

CHOOSING NOT CHEATING

'I didn't have a good week,' Andrea told me during an office visit. When she'd gone out to dinner, she told herself she wasn't going to dip into the bread basket. Andrea considers bread her weakness. But the bread came, and she couldn't resist it. She broke off a chunk of sourdough bread.

She would have felt okay if it had stopped there. But after that first bite of sourdough bread, she broke off another chunk. And then, perhaps because she was hungry or stressed, she had a third.

Somewhere between the second and third chunks of bread, she made the transition from feeling like she was in control to feeling that she'd blown her diet for that day. She told herself that she'd cheated, and she believed it. So she no longer felt good about herself. Since she felt like a failure anyway, she decided to have breaded veal cutlet followed by the Death by Chocolate cake for dessert. On the way home, she picked up some ice cream to snack on.

There's a good reason why I wage war on the concept of cheating: I simply don't believe that people cheat when they're hungry. If someone decides she has to have a brownie, I say, 'Go ahead, if you really want it. But make it a choice, not a cheat.'

'That brownie is 400 calories!' she replies. 'What's the difference whether you call it a 'cheat' or a 'choice'?'

The difference, I maintain, is logic. When you use logic to make the decision to eat some especially tempting, high-calorie food, you have the upper hand.

EATING WITH AWARENESS

Susan's evening started out like Andrea's, but the ending was quite different. Susan knows that she loves freshly baked breads and rolls.

She, too, went to a restaurant. When she saw the fresh, warm bread in the bread basket, she decided that she really wanted to have some, so she took a roll and enjoyed it.

I'm very familiar with Susan's history as a dieter. I know that in the past, taking that roll would have created a cascade effect. Instead of seeing the roll and deciding to eat and enjoy it, she would have picked at it – taking as little as possible, then taking some more, then finishing it. To someone with the mentality of a dieter, the roll is a trigger, and Susan would have finished the roll, then worked her way through the rest of the bread basket. She would have felt guilty the whole time because she was cheating.

Instead, Susan ordered fish and vegetables while she finished her roll. She enjoyed the whole meal – the high-calorie roll as well as the low-calorie meal – and came away from the table feeling good about herself.

WHAT'S THE DIFFERENCE?

The woman who *chose* the roll was listening to her feelings. Susan worked the roll into her 'diet' – if we use 'diet' to mean the standards that you set for yourself. Andrea, by contrast, didn't allow herself the awareness of what she was feeling. She tried to suppress the desire for bread. So when she finally gave in to that desire and ate the bread, not only did she mess up her eating plan but also she didn't feel good about herself.

> ## You should never have to live up to impossible standards

The problem? An impossible standard. If you love bread, there will be times when you want to have some. It's that simple. Right or wrong, self-image and self-worth for many people are very much related to what they're eating and how well they are sticking to their diets. The beauty of Food Awareness Training is that you're always choosing, never cheating. So you never have to feel like you're falling off the wagon.

MAKING YOUR DECISION

Obviously, you can't have every dessert in the world and still lose weight. But you do have some choices. You can pass over dessert, you can eat it, or you can choose one of many lower-calorie alternatives that may be just as satisfying. But whatever you do, recognise that the decision is up to you. Only choose the brownie if none of those lower-calorie options can possibly satisfy your desire for the flavour and texture of a brownie.

Making a conscious decision to enjoy something is very different from eating it and feeling like a failure. In the latter case, people often go on to an all-out binge, having decided that it doesn't matter since they've already blown the diet. Your attitude about what you're eating is as important a factor in how successful you'll be in weight loss as the calorie count of the food.

PERMISSION FROM THE DOCTOR

If you've been on diets before, you're probably wondering how I can be telling you that it is possible to eat until you feel satisfied and still lose weight – without weighing

Often, the lower-calorie choice is more delicious

yourself daily, measuring each portion or eating special weight-loss food products.

Many people find that they learn one thing immediately from our visual demonstrations: they can eat a whole lot more than they do now and still take in fewer calories.

And it's delicious food. Call me biased, but some of the foods that I recommend taste even better than foods that you're already eating. They're foods you can enjoy, foods you never realised were an option, possibly even new foods you've never tasted before. That's why many people come into my office and say that they don't feel like they're dieting.

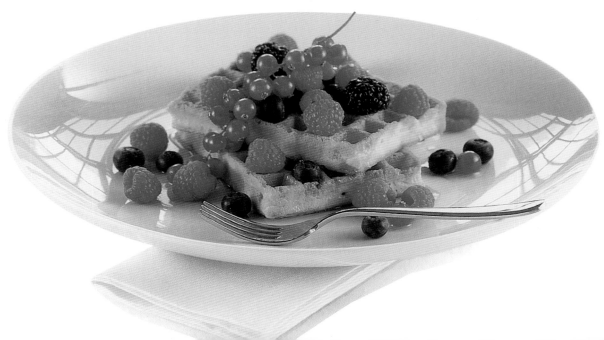

CALORIES AND WHERE THEY COME FROM

Nutrition is boring. Even nutritionists admit that. Fortunately, you don't need a course in nutrition to make Food Awareness Training work for you. We've taken a lot of the recent findings about nutrition and incorporated them in the food descriptions that are in this book. So while you're making your food choices, you can take note of the health benefits as well.

As you're making food choices, you will naturally lean towards foods that have lower calorie counts, since you want to lose weight. But in addition to this, I'd like to steer you towards foods that are high in nutritional value. It's a good way to make sure you're getting all the vitamins, minerals, fibre and protein that your body needs.

While I'm not going to give you a lecture here, I'd like to add a few notes to what you may have learned in school or picked up from your own reading – just enough to make nutrition awareness part of food awareness.

THE BIG PICTURE

Nutrients are divided into two basic categories, macronutrients and micronutrients. Macronutrients are food substances like protein, fat and carbohydrates that end up supplying us with calories.

I say 'end up', because calories are actually a measurement of how much energy is produced. For food to turn into energy, it has to be 'ignited' by the chemical processes in your body. A macronutrient has the potential to supply energy, and the actual production of energy is measured in calories.

Calories are calculated by measuring the amount of heat a food gives off when it is 'burned'.

If you've ever used an exercise bike that shows a digital readout of the calories you're burning, you've seen how they can go up in smoke when you're pedalling hard. Every action from breathing to scribbling a message on a postcard burns some calories. But, obviously, if you're pedalling an exercise bike, you are burning a lot more than you do when you scratch your chin.

Micronutrients are the sparks that help light the fire

Micronutrients are food components like vitamins and minerals. These help release energy from food, but supply no calories. This might surprise you, if you have always thought that vitamins give you energy. They don't. Certain vitamins give you better access to the macronutrients that supply the energy, but the vitamins themselves are not the fuel that feeds the fire. They're simply the sparks that help to ignite the energy-burning process.

What about water? Technically, it doesn't fit in either category. It's not a macronutrient, because it has no calories. And it's not a micronutrient, because it's neither a vitamin nor a mineral.

But we all know we need water to live. It's absolutely essential for digestion as well as many other bodily processes.

PROTEIN SOURCES

The nutrients – along with water – work like instruments in an orchestra. Each one has a specific task, but they work together to get the overall job done.

Proteins, among the macronutrients, are needed for growth and repair of tissues. The average person needs 45 to 55 grams of protein a day (although the average intake is between 60 to 90 grams). The requirement can be met with a bowl of bean soup and a seafood main course along with a good variety of vegetables and grains.

Protein is vital, but we should take care where we get it from

Each gram of protein has 4 calories. Typical high-protein foods include meat, fish, pulses, eggs, cheese and nuts, to mention just a few.

The reason that all protein foods don't have the same number of calories is because the fat and water content vary. That is why,

for example, most cheeses have 350 to 400 calories per 100 grams and most white fish have about 100 calories per 100 grams.

Cheese is a good example of a protein-rich food that's also a high-fat food. Yes, you get a high dose of protein from your favourite Cheddar. But along with it, you get saturated fat, which is the kind that contributes to heart disease and other problems.

As a result, we should turn to other, healthier, lower-calorie sources when we're looking for protein. Among the prime candidates are seafood and pulses like peas, beans and lentils.

The soyabean is a pulse that deserves special mention because of its health-promoting properties. That's why you'll see soya products pictured in this book. Any time you opt for any of the soya products that are currently available in the form of burgers, sausages or sliced meats or cheeses, you're choosing a high-protein, low-calorie food. These products, which are sold under various brand names, are increasingly available in supermarkets as well as health food stores.

LIQUID LUNCH

The phrase 'liquid lunch' once conjured up visions of Chief Executives downing their third martinis before heading back to the office. Today, it's more likely to refer to the meal-in-a-glass that serves as a lunch replacement for people on a diet.

Liquid meals are typically used by doctors to help sick patients gain nutrition. So it may seem logical to think that these meals are both healthy and convenient. Why not get our nutrition from a packet or a can?

There's a problem with this. While most of the weight-loss shakes contain a number of vitamins and minerals, they also contain substantial numbers of calories – as many as 250. Furthermore, they contain plenty of fat – up to 9 grams in some cases. What's more, most meal replacements provide neither fibre nor phytochemicals, the kind of thing you get best from eating vegetables and fruit.

If it's a milkshake you want, have one. If it's lunch you need, have a healthy meal.

COUNTING CARBS

Carbohydrates usually provide about half of your body's energy needs when you're resting or performing a low-level activity. About half the energy you burned last night while sleeping came from carbohydrate sources. And probably 50 per cent of the energy you're using right now, reading these words, comes from carbs. Carbohydrates are considered the energy nutrient, because your body can break them down and use them very quickly.

How much carbohydrate do you really need in your daily diet? For the average person, carbohydrate needs can be about 250 to 350 grams per day.

You've probably heard of runners or triathletes who eat lots of carbs before a big race; that's because they're going to be tapping a huge amount of that particular energy reservoir when they exercise hard. The requirements are a lot less, of course, if you hardly exercise.

> **In fat-free products, the fat is replaced with carbohydrates**

Sources of carbohydrates are all over the place. See that sugar bowl? Carbohydrates. Rice has carbohydrates. So do raisins, apples, spaghetti, popcorn, potatoes and biscuits.

SIMPLE AND COMPLEX

All carbs are not created equal. There are two basic types. The so-called 'simple carbohydrates' are the sugars. Cane sugar, any syrup, honey and the sugar in fruits are all simple carbohydrates. Then there are 'complex carbohydrates', or starches. Complex carbs include vegetables, such as potatoes, and grain products, such as bread, pasta and cereals.

Among the complex carbohydrates, there's a further distinction. Refined grain products such as white rice and white breads tend to suffer from processing. While these foods are being spruced up for delivery to our plates, they lose a lot of their hearty nutrients. Often, the packager takes steps to remedy that by enriching the food with iron and some B vitamins that are lost in processing.

Unrefined products – also complex carbohydrates – retain more of Mother Nature's supply of nutrients. Wholemeal bread and brown rice, for instance, have more protein, fibre, vitamins and minerals than their refined cousins. They also contain a whole category of beneficial nutrients that are often in short supply – the phytonutrients. These are health-promoting substances found in plants (aside from vitamins, minerals, and fibre) – see page 35.

CHECK THE INDEX?

Apart from the simple/complex division of carbohydrates, there's another way of categorising carbohydrate foods that you may have seen in some popular diet books: the glycaemic index, or GI.

The GI reflects the rate of entry of sugar into the bloodstream. In terms of weight loss, the slower the rate, the better. So the lower GI foods are considered better choices than the higher GI foods.

Many factors affect GI. Fibre, protein and fat content as well as the degree of processing of a food have a considerable effect on the glycaemic index. For example, wholemeal bread has a lower GI than white bread because of its fibre content. Sponge cake has a lower GI than plain, boiled rice because of its protein and fat content. And old-fashioned oats have a lower GI than instant oatmeal because they are less processed. Rice cakes happen to have a very high GI. Chocolate eclairs are relatively low!

You can see why discretion should be used when working with the GI. If you're encouraged to eat a wide range of fruits, vegetables, pulses and whole grains, that's fine. But if following the GI leads you to avoid potatoes, onions or carrots (which are high GI foods), that's not fine. And, please, go easy on the eclairs!

FATS IN THE FIRE

Every gram of fat has 9 calories. Compare that with the 4 calories in every gram of carbohydrate or protein, and you can see where fats get their ugly reputation. If you eat 1 gram of fat – that is, any kind of vegetable oil or animal fat – you're getting more than twice the calories you would get from 1 gram of carbohydrate or protein.

We need fats to survive. But researchers have had a hard time establishing how much fat we absolutely need in our diets.

The 'good', or unsaturated, fats are those that usually come from plants. They provide the essential fatty acids needed for good health. Unsaturated fats, studies have shown, have beneficial health effects: they help lower blood levels of low-density lipoproteins (LDLs), the 'bad cholesterol' contributing to artery-clogging plaque that clings to blood vessels and helps induce heart disease.

'Essential fatty acids' are fats that our bodies cannot make

Among the beneficial, unsaturated fats are soya oil, sunflower oil, olive oil and all other nut and seed oils. Flaxseed oil is the highest natural source of omega-3 fatty acids and is especially good for preventing health problems. And fish oil – especially the kind that comes from cold-water fish – is among the most beneficial of oils.

Any kind of oil has 120 calories per tablespoon

The 'bad', or saturated, fats are usually of animal origin. (Fish, high in omega-3 fatty acids, is the significant exception.) Bad fats tend to raise levels of LDL cholesterol and may increase the risk of certain cancers. Examples are chicken fat, beef fat, lard, butterfat and the fat found in eggs.

Another type of 'bad' fat is trans fat. This is the kind found in many margarines, solid cooking fat, and some fried food. It's formed when liquid oils are hydrogenated or hardened, or when they are heated to very high temperatures.

You will probably meet your requirement for essential fatty acids – unless, that is, you become fanatical about removing every trace of fat from your diet. By fanatical, I mean picking the few olives out of a Greek salad, being afraid to order grilled vegetables in a restaurant because they might be cooked in some form of oil, or choosing grilled sole from the menu, instead of salmon, even though you really don't like sole.

Remember, though, that all fats, whether 'good' or 'bad', are a very concentrated source of calories – 9 calories a gram. That's about 120 calories per tablespoon for any kind of oil.

So even if a fat is called 'good', like the fat in nuts, you can have too much of a good thing. At 600 to 700 calories per 100g, nuts come at a high cost.

MULTITASKING

Why do we need fats?

Like carbohydrates, fats are used for energy. But our need for fats goes beyond that. For instance, we require small amounts of essential fatty acids for efficient functioning of the immune system. The nervous system also needs fats.

Women need around 70 grams of fat a day and men need 95

And fats have been hired as ushers in the great theatre of our bodies. Many nutrients mix well with fat but not with water. If we're going to absorb these nutrients in our bodies – and get the benefits we need – fats have to help them make their way into our cells. We also need fat to help our bodies absorb some fat-soluble nutrients such as vitamins A, D, E and K.

And then there's the ice-cream effect. Fat contributes to a sense of satiety – that 'feeling full' sensation at the end of a meal. If you've cleaned your plate of the 23-vegetable special and you're still picking away at your dining partner's leftovers, maybe it's because you don't feel full. You want the gourmet ice cream at the end to achieve the 'Done!' feeling that you're after.

WHERE DOES THE LOW-FAT DIET GO WRONG?

Zero-fat diets are unhealthy. Why? Quite simply, because you need some fat in your diet if you want your brain, nerves and body to work.

But many people have heard that fat is the main culprit in weight gain. I have had patients who scrupulously followed a diet that prescribed 'No fat!' They conscientiously checked the fat grams on every food product they purchased. So, if they *still* gained weight, what went wrong?

Ardent dieters often make the mistaken assumption that only fat calories can make them gain weight. Fat-free food is not the answer, however.

Consider fat-free cakes and biscuits. You might assume that you can eat all you want. However, the refined carbohydrates in these foods can have more potential for weight gain than fat does.

I do not mean to suggest that people should necessarily avoid all low-fat products. Some low-fat dressings, sauces and frozen desserts make weight loss a lot easier than it used to be. It's the baked goods that are the culprits.

OVERFILLING ON FAT-FREE

Our brains communicate with our bellies in interesting ways. If a label says 'fat-free,' studies show, there's a good chance you'll eat *more* of that food – just as if you were giving yourself permission.

This conclusion is supported by a study at Pennsylvania State University where students were fed yoghurt products with a variety of fat content. When the students ate what they believed was a fat-free yoghurt, they ate more than normal at their next meal. But if they were told they were eating a high-fat yoghurt – and then followed it with a meal – they ended up eating *less* than usual.

In another study, researchers compared people eating fat-free crisps with those who ate ordinary crisps. True, the people eating fat-free crisps consumed less fat overall. But at the end of the day, they had consumed as many calories as the people who ate ordinary crisps. In terms of weight loss, there's no difference.

THE DELICACY WITH A DIAGNOSIS

Foie gras – literally, fatty liver – is produced by force-feeding geese or ducks until their livers are abnormally enlarged. In some countries its production has been banned because of its cruelty to animals.

Foie gras also has a huge number of calories – 450 per 100 grams to be precise. See for yourself: the health-destroying fat in a 100g morsel of this 'delicacy' is equivalent to five boxes of fast-food french fries and has the cholesterol equivalent of 17 tablespoons of pure lard.

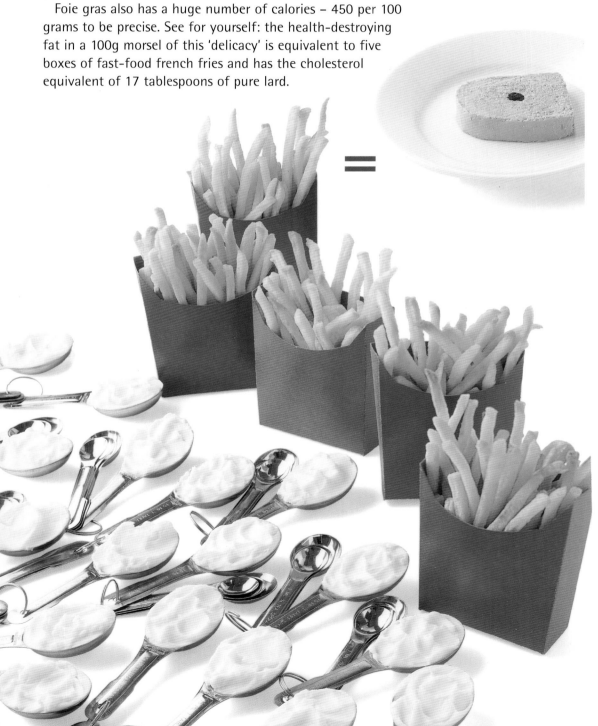

WHY CALORIES DO COUNT

When you consume more calories than you burn up, your body converts the unused carbohydrates, proteins or fats into body fat. This is why excess calories from any source can add interesting dimensions to your fat-absorbing stomach, hips and thighs.

> ## Women need around 2000 calories a day; men 2500

If we could just find a high-calorie, delicious food that would take 12 hours to eat, it wouldn't be such a threat to the waistline. The real 'problem foods' are the high-calorie gang that are quickly and easily consumed – such as pastries, chocolate bars, cake, crisps and biscuits. Not coincidentally, these are the villains that are usually considered 'fattening'. But they're not *necessarily* fattening. They're just easy to eat – and extraordinarily high in calories.

Regardless of how high they are in calories, you can have pastries, chocolate bars, cake, crisps and biscuits. But when you make the choice to eat these types of foods, you also need to figure out how you can eat low-calorie, filling foods as well.

WHAT A FRIEND IN FIBRE

You get fibre in your diet from fruit, vegetables, pulses and grains. Technically, fibre is a very complex carbohydrate. It is a structural component of plants.

Cellulose, which is an insoluble form of fibre, makes up the stems and skins of fruit and vegetables. There are also soluble forms found in pulses and oats. Since humans lack an enzyme to digest fibre, this type of food passes through our systems without being absorbed by the body.

Why is it important? We used to believe that fibre had one function only: to prevent constipation. Many people called it roughage – not a particularly appealing name for something that's travelling through the tender interior of your body.

Because of its somewhat unappealing reputation, if I say 'fibre' to many of my new patients, they associate it with food that isn't tasty, like raw bran. But there are many other, tasty foods are also high in fibre, ranging in variety from minestrone soup and marinated artichokes to vegetarian chilli, sweet potatoes, cherries and dried apricots.

We now know that fibre is far more than a constipation fighter. People on high-fibre diets reduce their risks of a whole range of different health problems, from high blood pressure and heart disease to digestive disorders and cancer.

High-fibre foods are bulky. They contribute to a sense of fullness because they take up a lot of space in your digestive tract. Since they may take up to 24 hours to pass through it, they can take the edge off your

> ## You can eat lots of fibre and consume very few calories

appetite (and thus reduce your calorie count) for as much as a day. Most also take a long time to chew, so they slow down your eating. All this means that you can fill up on fibre and still be eating less calories than you are actually using – which means that your body will have to use its existing energy stores.

High-fibre foods also tend to be excellent sources of nutrients. If you're eating a diet high in fibre – including fruit, vegetables and pulses – then you're eating a very healthy, low-calorie diet and not feeling hungry.

FIBRE FEASTS

Want to add fibre without any calorie penalty? From soup to snacks, the comparisons listed here show how you can fill up on fibre – and get lots of additional nutrients – without adding a single calorie. In fact, in most cases, you actually save calories when you go for the high-fibre choice. It's a win-win situation – and a feast of fibre.

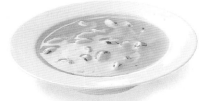 **VS**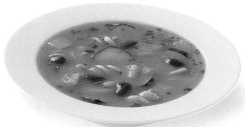

Chicken noodle soup (200ml)
0.5 grams fibre
150 calories

Vegetable soup (200ml)
5 grams fibre
110 calories

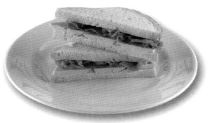 **VS**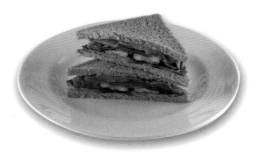

Turkey-on-white sandwich
1 gram fibre
290 calories

Grilled mediterranean vegetable sandwich
4 grams fibre
210 calories

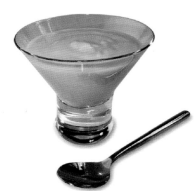 **VS**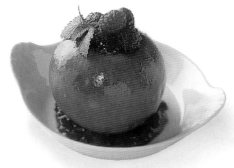

Fruit yoghurt (125g)
0 grams fibre
130 calories

Baked apple (200g) with raspberries
4 grams fibre
100 calories

GETTING THE NUTRIENTS YOU NEED

For a quick review of your vitamin and mineral needs, take a look at the table below.

Do you meet these requirements, given your daily diet? While you may eat a wide range of vegetables, fruit, pulses and grains, I would recommend that you also take a multivitamin supplement with minerals each day. A 'multi' provides an extra margin of safety. It simply ensures that you get all the recommended micronutrients that you need. Some vitamins – the water-soluble kind – cannot be stored in body for long periods, so they need to be replenished regularly.

The table below gives an average for the population. In fact, the recommended amounts are different for women and for men, and they change as we get older. What you need depends on your circumstances. Still growing?

RECOMMENDED DAILY ALLOWANCES

Finding out what vitamins and minerals you need can be confusing. Reference Nutrient Intakes (RNIs) or Recommended Dietary Intakes (RDIs) are the amounts of vitamin or mineral that will meet the requirements of almost every healthy person within a defined group. Below, you'll find recommendations for healthy adults – they may differ for children, older adults or pregnant women. If in doubt, consult your doctor.

Vitamin A/ Retinol
Required for healthy skin and eyesight. Found in fruit and vegetables containing carotene (such as carrots), oily fish and dairy products.
UK RNI for men: 700µg; for women: 600µg.
Australia/NZ RDI: 750 µg.
(Supplements and rich sources, such as liver, should be avoided by pregnant women.)

Vitamin B$_1$/ Thiamin
Needed to assist in the metabolism of fat, carbohydrate and alcohol. Found in fortified cereals, bread, vegetables, nuts, meat and pulses.
UK RNI for men: 1mg; for women: 0.8mg.
Australia/NZ RDI for men: 1.1mg; for women: 0.8mg.

Vitamin B$_2$/ Riboflavin
Needed for the metabolism of energy from fat, carbohydrate and protein. Found in fish, meat offal, dairy products, leafy vegetables and cereals.
UK RNI for men: 1.3mg; for women: 1.1mg.
Australia/NZ RDI for men: 1.7mg; for women: 1.2 mg.

Vitamin B$_3$/ Niacin
Required in digestive and nervous systems. Found in fish, vegetables, dairy products and cereals.
UK RNI for men: 17mg; for women: 13mg.
Australia/NZ RDI for men: 18–20mg; for women: 12–14mg.

Pantothenic acid/ Vitamin B$_5$
Converts fats, proteins and carbohydrates into energy. Found in eggs, fish, nuts and cereals.
No RNI.

Vitamin B$_6$/ Pyridoxine
For healthy blood and nervous system. Found in fish, meat, bananas, pulses and dairy products.
UK RNI for men: 1.4mg; for women: 1.2mg.
Australia/NZ RDI for men: 1.3–1.9mg; for women: 0.9–1.4mg.

Vitamin B$_{12}$/ Cyanocobalamin
Used in the formation of blood cells and genetic material, and in digestive / nervous systems. Only found in animal food sources or fortified foods.
UK RNI: 1.5µg. Australia/NZ RDI: 2µg.

Pregnant? Suffering from an illness? Even where you live and how your water supply is treated can affect your micronutrient needs. Your doctor may have a particular reason for prescribing something extra. (For instance, you might be prescribed folic acid before or during pregnancy, calcium for osteoporosis or vitamin E for heart disease.)

I am opposed, however, to megadoses of vitamins or minerals. If you're eating a healthy and varied diet and taking an adequate multivitamin, it's a pretty safe bet that you're getting all the micronutrients you need. In fact, manufacturers in many countries are required to fortify flour with calcium and margarine with fat-soluble vitamins, and many soft drinks and breakfast cereals are also fortified with vitamins and minerals – so you will get a lot of these micronutrients from your food.

Folic acid/ Folate
Used in the formation of blood cells and genetic material. Found in meat, fortified cereals, breads, eggs, pulses, nuts, green vegetables. **UK/Australia/NZ RNI: 200µg** (This figure differs for pregnancy.)

Vitamin C
Required for healthy skin, teeth, gums and blood vessels; aids the absorption of iron. Found in a variety of fruit and vegetables. **UK RNI: 40mg. Australia/NZ RDI for men: 40mg; for women: 30mg.**

Vitamin D/ Cholecalciferol
Required for absorption of phosphorus and calcium. The main source is sunlight. Also found in breakfast cereals, eggs and oily fish. **UK RNI: 10µg** (There is no RNI for adults under 65.) **Australia/NZ No RDI.**

Vitamin E/ Tocopherols
Protects body tissues. Found in dark green leafy vegetables, vegetable oils, fish, nuts and pulses. **UK** Safe intakes for men: 4mg; for women: 3mg. **Australia/NZ RDI** for men: 10mg; for women: 7mg.

Vitamin K/ Phylloquinone
Needed for normal blood clotting. Found in green, leafy vegetables, eggs and oats. No RNI.

Calcium
For healthy bones and teeth. Sources include dairy products, tofu, bony fish and dried fruit. **UK RNI: 700mg. Australia/NZ RDI: 800mg.**

Iodine
Used in regulating the thyroid gland. Found in fatty fish, seafood, eggs, iodised salt and dairy products. **UK RNI: 140µg. Australia RDI** for men: 150µg; for women: 120µg. **NZ RDI 200µg.**

Iron
For red blood cells. Sources include red meat, offal, oily fish, pulses and fortified cereals. **UK RNI** for men: 8.7mg; for women: 14.8mg. **Australia/NZ RDI** for men: 7mg; for women: 12–16mg.

Magnesium
Used in energy production, healthy bones and the nervous system. Found in whole-grains, nuts, tofu, beans, meat and fish. **UK RNI** for men: 300mg; for women: 270mg. **Australia/NZ RDI** for men: 320mg; for women: 270mg.

Phosphorus
Needed for energy production, healthy teeth and bones. Found in all foods. **UK RNI: 550mg. Australia/NZ RDI: 1000mg.**

Zinc
Used by the immune system and in growth. Found in meat, dairy products, fish and pulses. **UK RNI** for men: 9.5mg; for women: 7mg. **Australia/NZ RDI: 12mg.**

WHAT ABOUT MIRACLE FORMULAS?

Not only am I opposed to multidoses of certain vitamins, I am also opposed to some of the over-the-counter remedies for weight loss.

It's important for every consumer to realise that substances sold as natural food supplements are not subject to the same regulations as prescription drugs. But weight-loss supplements – sold under a host of inviting names – can be just as potent as prescription medicines.

My objections to weight-loss medications are based on issues of safety and efficacy. Here are my views:

■ There is no standardised means of extraction. The quantity of the active substance might vary widely from one product to the next, even though both labels bear the same description. Also, impurities may be present.

■ Some remedies may be utterly useless, which defrauds the public.

■ Some may have toxic effects either alone or in combination with other drugs that people may be using.

■ There may be insufficient or no warnings about usage or dosage.

WHERE 'NATURAL' IS NOT ALL

What is unfortunate is that people believe readily available herbs and herbal formulas are not medicines. Many people think, 'They're just herbs', and because they are 'natural', they are perceived as safe and healthy. This could not be further from the truth.

Some of the most potent, toxic substances known to mankind are natural. Just because something is herbal or derived from a plant doesn't mean it's safe. People are often drawn to these products because they get a feeling of control over their own health care. As a doctor, I am concerned that a person's response to these substances is not monitored. Some of these natural remedies can have profound effects on body functions such as heart rate and blood pressure.

FUNCTIONAL FOODS: HEALTH WEAPON OR MARKETING FAD?

Cholesterol-reducing chocolate bars? Mood-lightening pasta? With the functional, or 'prescription' food industry growing every year, such fantasies are increasingly possible. Functional foods go beyond 'fortified' foods – those containing extra vitamins or minerals – to add a range of putative nutrients to a variety of food products. The idea that we can improve our health by eating certain products is an attractive one to consumers and manufacturers alike.

> **Functional foods claim to have health benefits**

Since many of the ingredients are natural, functional foods strike consumers as being healthy. Are they?

Not necessarily. Some functional foods may provoke allergic reactions. Some may not combine well with any medicines you might be taking. Some may have side effects. Besides, the food label won't tell you how much you should eat or for how long you should eat it – the kind of information that is required for 'real' medicines.

Although manufacturers of functional foods assert only that their products affect body function rather than fight disease, European Union guidelines state that their claims must be based on sound and valid scientific evidence.

DRESSING DOWN

Researchers report that salad dressing is a major source of fat in the dieter's diet. This is especially the case for women under the age of 50 who eat a lot of salad – no doubt on the theory that it's good for them. So it is, as long as you watch the dressing.

A ladle of salad dressing may contain as much as 48 grams of fat and 450 calories. Commercial dressings are primarily fat, with 85 per cent of their calorie content derived from oil. Instead, try the fat-free or low-fat commercial dressings. Or, when you're at home or at the salad bar, make your own lower-fat vinegar-and-oil dressing, making it go further by adding lemon or tomato juice and a range of condiments such a ketchup, salsa, relish and mustard. In restaurants, ask for low-fat dressing or for oil and vinegar 'on the side'.

PHYTO FACTS

In addition to the vitamins and minerals, there is another class of substances known as phytochemicals whose role in human nutrition is just becoming clear. Phytochemicals seem to have an important role in the prevention of diseases. While these phytochemicals have no direct effect on weight loss, a person who is eating the type of healthy diet I recommend – rich in fruit, vegetables and pulses – will be getting a good dose of phytochemicals to decrease the risk of heart disease, cancer and other diseases.

Phytochemical Family	Food Sources
Allyl sulphides	Onions, garlic, leeks, chives
Isoflavones	Soyabeans (tofu, soya milk)
Isothiocyanates	Cruciferous vegetables (brocoli, Brussels sprouts, cabbage, cauliflower)
Phenolic acids (ellagic acid, ferulic acid)	Tomatoes, citrus fruits, carrots, whole grains, nuts
Polyphenols, flavonoids	Black and green tea, apples, onions, citrus fruits, carrots, broccoli, cabbage, soya products, parsley, tomatoes, aubergine, peppers, berries
Saponins	Beans and pulses
Terpenes (perilyl alcohol, limonene)	Cherries, citrus fruit peel

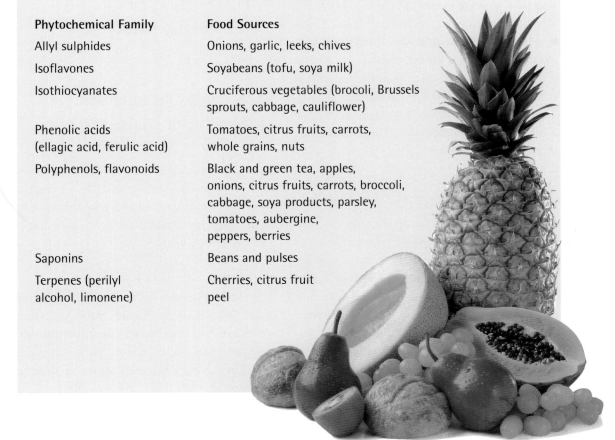

DIET MYTHS EXPLODED

If you thought this was a 'diet book' when you picked it up, I hope you're now convinced otherwise.

As you can tell, I simply don't believe that diets can help you lose weight permanently. They rely too heavily on prescribing exactly why, when, what or how much you should eat. As I've realised from working with people who really do lose weight – and do keep it off – we simply need to change our relationship with food so we make mindful decisions about what we eat.

But diets abound, and so do diet books. Celebrity-authored diet books are all the rage. High-protein, low-carb diets are popular. And every health magazine seems to feature a new 'quick-fix' diet.

So, what's wrong with these diets? That's the question that people ask me over and over again. After all, they're supposed to 'work', and if people go on a diet, and it doesn't work for them, they feel as if they're at fault.

I don't care if you've been on one diet or a hundred. If a diet hasn't worked for you, that's not your fault. In the long run, diets don't work.

HISTORY REPEATING ITSELF

Changing your relationship with food is the primary focus of the weight-loss programme you're about to undertake, but that isn't the only thing that should change. You'll also want to alter or abandon a considerable number of common misconceptions about losing weight.

The subject goes back as much as half a century. That's when the diet game really seems to have got going, and it marks the first of many phases that dieting has gone through since that time. Each phase of enthusiasm was driven by what dieters were told was a newly discovered truth or a newly invented magic bullet. This time, they were told, the new plan was really going to make a difference!

THE COUNTING CRAZE

Back in the post-war period of the 1950s, suburban lifestyles were emerging as the norm, and thin was in. Calorie-counting devices were all the rage. All you had to do was spin a wheel or click a counter to see how many calories that apple or plate of spaghetti was costing you. Then you'd add up the calories for the meal or the day. And finally, you'd check your intake against a set formula.

The formula was based on the 'fact' that to lose a pound (455g) of fat, you must give up 3500 calories. Therefore, if you ate 500

> **A simple formula told you how much you would lose**

fewer calories than normal for 7 consecutive days (7 x 500), you would lose nearly a pound. We now know this is too simplistic an assumption, but at the time, it was the Gospel for calorie counters.

FAT IS THE ENEMY

The next big trend was fat restriction. By the early 1980s, the buzz was that all fats were bad, and the goal was to consume as few as possible. Carbohydrate calories, by contrast, were considered good – that is to say, it was assumed they wouldn't adversely affect weight loss.

People were encouraged to eat carbs to their hearts' desire, so long as they cut out fat. The result was a boom in the sale and consumption of pasta, bagels, breads and fat-free biscuits and cakes. Another result was that many people gained lots of weight.

By the late 1980s and early 1990s, the experts were taking a closer look at carbohydrates. Wasn't there a significant difference, they asked, between simple carbohydrates such as sugar and the complex carbohydrates found in starchy foods?

According to the new thinking, complex carbohydrates were better for us than simple carbohydrates because they took longer to break down and were less likely to be stored as fat.

FROM UNREFINED TO GLYCAEMIC INDEX

During the mid 1990s, it became clear that the distinction between simple and complex carbohydrates wasn't so clear. You also had to know whether the carbohydrate was refined or unrefined. Down went dieters' consumption of such refined carbohydrates as white rice, most pasta and white breads like bagels and sourdough. Up went the intake of unrefined carbs such as whole-grain pastas and breads along with lots of starchy vegetables.

In the late 1990s, the glycaemic index became the rage. This index reflects the rate at which sugar enters into the bloodstream. For purposes of weight loss, the slower the rate of entry the better. Foods with a high glycaemic index include white rice, white potatoes, beetroot and carrots. These were suddenly considered off-limits. Sweet potatoes and whole grains – foods with a low glycaemic index – suddenly filled dieters' plates.

FOOD COMBINING

Everyone would like a formula that's guaranteed to work, and some people have gone out on a limb to provide just that. Among the most creative and least credible of these fomulas is 'food combining'. It is based on the notion that because different nutrients are digested at different rates, the 'wrong' combination of foods can lead to poor digestion and increased fat storage.

This is nonsense, and those who promote it as a method of weight loss must have been absent the day the rest of us learned about nutrition in school. Food that is not digested cannot be absorbed into the bloodstream and therefore cannot be deposited as body fat.

But people do lose weight on these programmes. In fact, a number of people have told me that they met someone or talked to someone who actually lost several pounds. No doubt. But the person lost weight because he or she took in less carbohydrate and/or fewer calories, not because she didn't mix protein and carbs at the same meal.

GIMMICK GAMES

'Fat-burning foods' are another myth of the diet game. There are those who maintain that grapefruit burns fat, or that vinegar or lemon juice melts it away. But no food burns fat. Maybe it's the tart taste of these foods that inspires people to this wishful image, but it simply is not so.

> ## Exercise burns fat; food does not

Remember the cabbage soup diet? Thousands of people tried it. Then there was the watermelon diet. And the ice-cream diet – yes, there was one. All of these gimmick diets have a similar theme. They restrict your intake of total calories. When your eating is restricted to one or two foods, you tend to eat less just because it's so boring to eat the same thing all the time.

So naturally, for a week or two, you will be thrilled with what the scales tell you. But the large loss registered by the scales is not totally a loss of fat. Instead, it's mainly due to a loss of fluid — in part, because you've reduced your intake of sodium and/or carbohydrate — and it's temporary.

Advocates of gimmick diets typically recommend that you stay on them for 1 or 2 weeks only. They're not very healthy, and they probably won't continue to work after 2 weeks. The drop on the scales will taper off, the lost fluids will come back and you'll regain the weight you lost.

Besides, by the second week, you'll be so bored with the monotony of what you're eating — not to mention with your low energy and generally lack-lustre feeling — that you won't continue to follow the regime.

BUST THAT SUGAR HABIT

The 'Sugar Busters' diet is based exclusively on the glycaemic index. To ensure that the diet favours low-glycaemic-index foods, the authors of the Sugar Busters diet exclude all refined carbohydrates. You can, however, consume liberal amounts of animal proteins

> ## Supposedly, the lower the glycaemic index the better

and fats. This alone detracts from the healthiness of the Sugar Buster diet.

In addition, some of the food recommendations don't always make sense. For example, you are not allowed to have

carrots, a ripe banana or a piece of watermelon. But chocolate bars are fine as long as they contain 70 per cent cocoa, and ice cream is welcome as long as it has a very

> ## Many 'diets' allow a high consumption of protein and fat

high fat content. Commercial peanut butter, on the other hand, is not permitted because of its very small quantity of added sugar.

My quarrel with Sugar Busters is that the authors let you eat an entire cow, pig or deer if you want to, but they don't let you flavour it with teriyaki sauce or accompany it with pickle or coleslaw. The moral is, you can have as much protein and fat as you can stomach, but don't even think about the second half of that artichoke!

'SOMERSIZING'

Suzanne Somers recommends a form of food combining that she has dubbed 'Somersizing'. Somers has figured out that since protein, fats and carbohydrates are digested at different rates, combining them 'improperly,' as she puts it, will halt digestion. Poorly digested food, she goes on to claim, is more likely to be stored as body fat.

There's just one problem with this neatly logical explanation. It has no basis in fact. Undigested food cannot be absorbed from the intestine into the bloodstream, let alone stored as fat.

Yet on the basis of this incorrect assertion, Somers prescribes a stringent eating plan. She specifies that fat can be eaten together with protein, but not with carbohydrates. Fruit must be eaten by itself as a separate meal, while foods containing sugar and white flour must be eliminated.

Some odd discrepancies crop up in the Somersizing programme. Somers puts banana, pumpkin and winter squash on the same list as white flour. So these foods are to be eliminated from your diet. She lists beetroot and carrots in the same category as white sugar, so they have to go as well!

Somers also wants you to eliminate what she calls 'bad combo' foods from your diet. These are foods that contain small amounts of carbohydrate in addition to protein and fat and that therefore cannot be neatly placed

To say that fruit can 'cause' fat is downright absurd

into any other category. Bad combo foods include nuts, olives, tofu and soya milk.

Ironically, the amount of carbohydrate in a serving of tofu or olives, for example, is insignificant – ½ to 2 grams – and is much lower than the amount of carbohydrate found in many of the foods Somers allows. As these examples and many others suggest, her 'bad combo foods' are very healthy. Many nutritionists wish people would actually eat more of the foods that are on Somers's banned list.

The misinformation in the book is sometimes startling. The glycaemic index, Somers tells us, 'rises corresponding to the level of hyperglycaemia caused by eating carbohydrates. The higher the glycaemic index, the higher the level of hyperglycaemia.'

This is just one example of many mis-statements. Hyperglycaemia, or too much sugar in the blood, is usually seen in diabetics. Normal individuals maintain their blood sugar ranges regardless of what they've eaten. The glycaemic index of a food – not of a person – does not change and is not influenced by high blood sugar, low blood sugar, or anything else in the body.

To put this another way, if Somers were correct in her assumptions, everyone's blood sugar would be off the charts. We'd have sugar crystals in our veins after eating a rice cake or a carrot, both of which have a high-glycaemic index.

I think my favourite, however, is the author's claim that fruit is not a healthy choice for dessert because 'if you mix fruit with other foods, it can lose its nutritional benefit'. What's more, says Somers, fruit 'spoils in the stomach (and). . . can trap the energy of other foods and cause unnecessary storage of fat'.

Somers suggests, instead, various rich cakes and pies that make wonderful desserts, in her view. Recipes for these desserts are included in the book. There's nothing wrong with cakes and pies, but to say that fruit can 'lose its nutritional benefit' or 'trap the energy of other foods' is not just wrong, it's ridiculous.

THE CONTROL ISSUE

Have you always associated weight loss with self-control? I hope I can convince you otherwise.

Contrary to conventional wisdom, control is not the sure path to weight loss. In fact, control is the enemy. It suggests that someone *wants* to eat a particular food but refuses to do it with a mighty effort of will.

This kind of control goes hand in hand with deprivation, which ultimately spells trouble. There will be a breakdown of willpower sooner or later. When you lose weight by obsessively controlling what you eat rather than by making choices, you're very likely to regain that weight again as soon as you 'lose control'.

THE ATKINS APPROACH

As we enter a new millennium, we find ourselves in a new phase of diet wisdom. Today, the prevailing trend is an emphasis on protein consumption. High-protein, low-carbohydrate diets now ride the crest of the popularity wave.

According to the late Dr Robert C. Atkins, your fastest route to weight loss is paved with lots of protein and fat – and no carbohydrates. The Atkins diet is based on the theory that if you restrict carbohydrate, the body will turn to its fat stores for energy.

What the Atkins diet does is simple: it puts the dieter into a state of ketosis. Ketones are substances that form when fat is broken down for energy but not completely burned or metabolised.

If you subscribe to this reasoning, then the presence of ketones – in the urine 'proves' that body fat is being broken down.

There are two things wrong with this. Firstly, biochemists are not certain that the ketones in the blood or urine are products of broken-down body fat or of dietary fat – that is, of the high fat content of the Atkins diet. Secondly, ketones are not normally present in the blood or urine. They are typically seen in uncontrolled diabetes or starvation.

It's probably safe to say that a mild degree of ketosis, from time to time, won't hurt you, but we aren't sure about the long-term effects of being in a constant state of ketosis. If you have type 1 diabetes, are pregnant or thinking about becoming pregnant or have gout or a family history of gout, you should *absolutely not* be on a ketogenic diet.

Another possible effect of the Atkins diet is its lowering of the brain chemical serotonin, one of the body's main controllers of mood and appetite. Serotonin needs some carbohydrate to keep on working. It's no wonder, therefore, that people on very low carb diets often feel down, depressed, irritable or all of the above.

What's more, people invariably find that once they 'go off' the low-carb diet, they virtually binge on carbohydrate foods. Whether low serotonin levels are to blame for this effect is not yet proven, but they tend to show up in Atkins dieters.

Will you lose weight on the Atkins diet? Probably. But, apart from ketosis – which can be dangerous – and possibly low serotonin levels – is the Atkins diet healthy?

Not in our view – and not in the view of most health care professionals. Our concern, of course, is with the high intake of animal protein and fat that the Atkins diet entails, which can increase the risk of many diseases. Also, the diet stringently restricts carbohydrates – every food, every meal, every day. Because of the strict limits on fruit, grains and many vegetables, it's nearly impossible to meet your needs for vitamins, minerals and

A DAY OF ATKINS DINING

What follows is a day in the life of an Atkins dieter. In our view, this is a diet that will catch up with you sooner rather than later, as you add back the pounds and put a heavy burden on your body's functioning. For all meals, there are no limits on portion size.

Breakfast: Fried eggs, sugarless sausages

Lunch: Salad with ham, cheese, chicken, egg and sugar-free dressing

Dinner: Prawn cocktail with mustard and mayonnaise dressing, clear consommé, steak, green salad with sugar-free dressing, diet jelly with whipped double cream

fibre on the Atkins diet without resorting to supplements.

Certainly, some of the effects of the high-fat, high-protein diet can be mitigated if you get most of your protein from such foods as fish and soya products, and most of your fat from the likes of olive or rapeseed oil or nuts, for example. But let's face it: the vast majority of Atkins dieters are there for the meat, cheese and butter. Who can blame them? On a diet that is this restrictive, there needs to be some compensation.

ARE YOU A CARB ADDICT?

Most health professionals, myself included, will tell you that you can't be addicted to a nutrient like carbohydrate. Sure, there may be some superficial similarities between the thoughts and behaviours of drug addicts and dieters/bingers. But the differences between them are substantial – and fundamental. Yet Doctors Richard F. Heller and Rachael F. Heller maintain that people who are 'hooked' on carbs can get 'unhooked' somehow.

They propose a diet that's based on the intricacies of insulin secretion. It requires two meals a day to consist of protein and low-carb vegetables – very much like the diet proposed by Dr Atkins. Unlike Dr Atkins, however, the Hellers give you one meal a day when you can eat anything you want, as long as the meal is consumed within a 60-minute time frame. The Hellers' diet also allows you to eat whatever amount of food you want, both at the two low-carbohydrate meals and at the 'reward' meal.

This low-carbohydrate diet is easier to follow than the Atkins diet, and it can be nutritionally adequate – depending, to a great extent, on what you eat at your 'reward' meal. But the liberal use of meat, poultry and dairy products can put you at risk of diseases such as cancer and osteoporosis. And while you may indeed lose weight – depending on your calorie needs and your prior eating habits – your choice of foods at the 'reward' meal will play an important role in how much you lose and how long you keep it off.

THE POWER OF PROTEIN

Doctors Michael Eades and Mary Dan Eades, in their book *Protein Power*, recommend another kind of low-carb, high-protein diet. They allow you a daily ration of 25 to 30 grams of carbohydrate, to be distributed evenly throughout the day. Obviously, that requires very stringent portion control on fruit, grains and vegetables.

The authors assure dieters that there is no need to not worry about fat. They even put butter on their list of 'good fats'. They also urge you to be as liberal as you want with

High intake of animal foods increases risk of heart disease

steak, eggs, bacon and the like without fear of heart disease. The reason, say the authors, is that the liver will not manufacture cholesterol from these foods unless they're eaten together with starch or sugar. That's a dubious proposition.

Protein Power also contends that vegetarian diets are monotonous – an ironic claim given that every meal in the book can be prepared with the tasty vegetarian products available today. Moreover, the authors claim that 'the most serious deficiency that vegetarians face is protein malnourishment'. That's not ironic – it's untrue. Studies have long proved that soya protein, which makes up most of the meat substitutes available today, is of equal value to animal protein.

ZONE MASTERY

The Zone is a rigid diet plan by Barry Sears, PhD. Virtually everything about this diet is carefully calculated and regulated. Dr Sears tells people when to eat, what to eat and how much. Your protein, carbohydrate and fat allowances are carefully apportioned in 'blocks'. You pick foods from those blocks and make sure they're distributed among three meals and two snacks every day.

The proportional relationships among protein, carbohydrate and fat are predetermined. Those proportions must remain the same whether you're having a full meal or just a snack. No food exceptions are allowed, and there are no concessions to mood, circumstance or degree of hunger.

The Zone is carefully reasoned, and it builds upon what scientists know about the biochemistry of weight loss. The diet is designed to create a hormonal balance that will maximise fat loss while supposedly keeping your energy level up and your hunger level down. Because the Zone is low in calories and fairly low in carbohydrates, you are likely to lose weight on it. And it can be healthy, although a lot depends on which options you select from your daily 'blocks'.

The downsides is that it is so rigidly controlled. You can never have just a piece of fruit on the Zone, or a bowl of pasta. You would have to have a specific portion of each, and you would be required to eat it together with a well-regulated portion of protein and portion of fat. It may indeed work for some people, but it does so at the sacrifice of your relationship with food. Look at the sample meal (below, left) and you'll see why.

DIETING PILLS

Weight-loss products abound on the shelves of chemists, health food shops and even supermarkets. They contain a range of ingredients – some of them utterly ineffective, some completely unsafe. Some ingredients do decrease appetite or increase fat loss, but their long-term safety has not been established.

What makes these products especially troublesome is that they are sold without prescription. Some of them can be nearly as potent as prescription drugs and are potentially dangerous. Nor is it known if the weight that's taken off comes back, as is the case with most diets.

No weight-loss product is recommended in this book. As to the ingredients in these products, here's a partial rundown, starting with the 'fat blockers'.

Over-the-counter fat blockers prevent a certain amount of dietary fat from being absorbed from the intestine. In controlled studies, chitosan – a fat blocker made from the exoskeletons of shellfish – did seem to have some effect on weight loss. However, in other clinical studies, large doses of

---

A MEAL IN THE SNACK ZONE

The meal and snack below are representative of the portion sizes you must restrict yourself to on the Zone diet. At every meal and snack, the ratio among the three food groups – protein, carbohydrate and fat – must be 40-30-30. Food for each of the groups is apportioned in 'blocks'.

Zone meal

3 blocks protein	90g chicken
3 blocks carbohydrate	¾ pitta bread
3 blocks fat	½ tbsp peanut butter

Zone snack

1 block protein	30g lean meat
1 block carbohydrate	⅓ pear
1 block fat	1 macadamia nut

chitosan caused a sharp drop in the blood levels of vitamin E, intensified the loss of calcium from bones and resulted in the loss of other minerals. So I'm reserving judgement on this one until more is known about its long-term effects.

Probably the most publicised of the pills with a promise was Fen-phen. Fen-phen is the shorthand name for a combination of drugs that was first hailed as the solution for weight control, then banned because of health concerns. For popular consumption, prescription Fen-phen was 'replaced' by a herbal equivalent – a combination of ma huang (ephedra) and St John's wort.

This combination, however, also raised health concerns. St John's wort is a mood enhancer and antidepressant that affects the brain chemical serotonin, which influences both mood and appetite. As for ma huang, some studies indicate that it does increase fat loss. But a number of fatalities have been associated with its use, and I strongly caution against the use of herbal Fen-phen products.

PILL PROMISES

Here are some of the other popular products that promise weight loss in a pill. Some of these are not available over the counter but are available on the internet.

Cassia (senna) and garcinia (camboge): These act as laxatives and can be dangerous, particularly for people with a history of intestinal obstruction or inflammatory intestinal disease.

Cellasene: A very expensive treatment made of herbs, seeds, fish oil and soya lecithin. Dangerous for pregnant women, and for those with thyroid conditions or on blood thinners.

Chromium picolinate: Thought to play a role in insulin metabolism, chromium is essential in trace amounts, but can be toxic in large doses. It does not change body composition and may adversely affect the body's use of iron.

Conjugated linoleic acid (CLA): A mixture of fatty acids that form in the intestines of cattle, CLA has no effect on overweight human adults.

Hawthorn, ginseng and ginkgo biloba: These have no proven effect on weight loss.

Hydroxycitric acid (HCA): HCA inhibits the enzyme that turns citric acid to fat. It also has a laxative effect and has been shown to be toxic in animal studies. As for weight loss in humans, HCA has no consistent effect.

L-arginine, L-ornithine and L-lysine: These amino acids are said to help metabolize fat, but no studies have proven any measurable effect.

L-carnitine: An amino acid that plays a role in fat metabolism. Some overweight people may have low levels of L-carnitine, but supplements have not been proven to affect weight loss.

Orlistat (Xenical): This drug, which inhibits fat absorption, is available by prescription.

Phenylpropanalomine (PPL): This suppresses appetite by increasing the level of a brain chemical called dopamine. Dangerous if you have heart, thyroid or kidney disease, high blood pressure or if you're pregnant.

Pyruvate: Made in the body and found in some foods, pyruvate has an insignificant effect on weight loss. Its long-term safety is unknown.

Reductil (Sibutramine): An appetite supressant that is available on prescription.

WHAT'S WRONG WITH DIETS?

We've already looked at the most prominent of the current crop of diet books. For each, we answer two questions: 'Is the diet healthy?' and 'Will you lose weight by following it?'

By 'a healthy diet', we mean two things. The diet should first supply adequate amounts of protein, vitamins and minerals.

A diet should contain adequate amounts of essential nutrients

Secondly, it should decrease the risk of such diet-related diseases as cancer, heart disease, diabetes and osteoporosis.

During the last two decades, research has made it clear that the healthiest diet is one that includes a variety of vegetables, fruit, whole grains and protein from vegetable rather than from animal sources. Despite these findings, most of the books focus on carbohydrate restriction while allowing liberal quantities of animal protein and fats.

It's important not to lump together all protein foods or all fats. There is a distinction between animal and vegetable protein – between beans or veggie-burgers, for example, and cheese or steak. Similarly, not all fats are equal. Butter and bacon should not be equated with olive oil and nuts. Fish is probably the only animal food worth including in your diet because it's a good source of essential fatty acids. But even if fish is a good source of these 'good fats', nuts, seeds and vegetable oils are probably the best sources.

CORRECTING OUR COURSE

Over the years, as we've moved through various diet fads and phases, I've noticed that many of the assumptions behind these diets

do have merit. Consuming fewer calories will certainly help you lose weight. Restricting fats, within reason, is probably a good health move. Eating more protein-packed foods and fewer carbohydrate-heavy foods may lead to weight loss.

But if these pearls of diet wisdom aren't lies, they're not the whole truth, either. And around them have swirled a maelstrom of assumptions, assertions and assurances that have been repeated so often they've been accepted into the dieter's canon of laws.

So before you eat another thing, let's cut through the fuzz and put the whole picture into sharp focus. Let's look at food. You can't stop eating, and you don't want to. So let's work out how to make choices about the food you eat.

HOW SWEET IT IS

Desserts and sweets are invariably the first things people believe they must give up when they are trying to lose weight. Sweets, biscuits and cakes are seen as obvious taboos. But the fact is, you don't have to give them up at all. In fact, it's unnatural to do so. A liking for sweet foods is ingrained into our basic

Liking sweet things is a fundamental human instinct

survival instincts. Deprive yourself of sweet things for too long, and when you finally do allow yourself some, you tend to run amok. Then it's blow-out time, as you binge on your favourite dessert, and after the blow-out comes the guilt, the regret, the self-recrimination – and more sweets.

Instead of depriving yourself of sweet treats, turn to the lower-calorie sweets and desserts that are pictured in the food demonstrations and described in the Anytime List on page 138. There are plenty of low-calorie choices you can eat with enjoyment without undermining your weight-loss effort.

HOW ABOUT A DRINK?

What about my evening cocktail? What about my glass of wine with dinner? Sometimes, this is the first thing people ask me.

Well, awareness is the key when you're making this choice. The first thing to be aware of is that studies have suggested that alcohol may actually increase appetite. What is almost certain is that it decreases your resistance and can tend to muddle the decision-making process. In a study, researchers alternated between giving alcoholic and non-alcoholic aperitifs to a group of men and women lunchers over a 7-day period. On the days when the group drank alcohol, they ate faster, ate more, ate for a longer time, became 'full' later, and kept on eating even after they had reached satiety.

Certainly, the alcohol prompted the people in the study to eat more and eat faster. Perhaps it also made them throw caution to the wind.

Since your food choices are the key to your weight loss, if alcohol tends to put you in a devil-may-care mood, that's something you ought to recognise. If you find that a bowl of peanuts at the bar disappears in the blink of an eye when you're meeting the gang for a few rounds of beer, you may want to keep an eye on your intake. Here's some overall advice for those times when drinks are being served:

■ Choose soda or mineral water with a twist of lime or lemon for your first drink or two, because the first drink goes down so quickly. Only then move on to a glass of wine or a long drink.

■ Order a bottle of mineral water to come to the table when the bottle of wine is ordered. After that, alternate your glasses: first water, then wine. You'll pace your drinking.

ACCOUNTING FOR TASTE

Tastebuds, filled with nerve fibres, are on your tongue, on the roof of your mouth, inside your cheeks, even in your throat. Complex interactions take place within and among the tastebuds and brain both to evaluate flavours – sweet, sour, bitter, salty – and measure the level of savouriness. What's more, senses in your mouth and nasal system augment the tasting process, which is why you 'can't taste a thing' when you have a cold.

A nerve connecting the brain, nose and mouth is another player in the taste game; it detects spicy irritants in such foods as hot chilli peppers, the cool sensations of foods like mint and the carbonation effect in certain beverages.

What's more, hot food is easier to taste than cold food – firstly, because it gives off more vapour, and secondly, because heat actually increases the intensity of sweet or bitter flavours, while cold diminishes it.

So keep these facts in mind when you're enjoying good food. Your tastebuds need looking after. And if they get what they want, your stomach will in turn feel very satisfied.

COOKED VERSUS RAW

Some people are under the impression that cooked vegetables have more calories than raw vegetables. In a sense, they're right: a plateful of raw spinach has fewer calories than a plateful of cooked spinach. That's because when spinach cooks, it shrinks, and you can therefore pack more onto a plate.

But that's measuring by volume. By weight, the calories are the same whether you eat your spinach cooked or raw. And the same is true with broccoli, courgettes, carrots and any other vegetable that can be eaten either way.

I am constantly telling my patients that it makes good sense to eat their vegetables cooked as well as raw — as long as they are not so over-cooked that all the goodness has been lost. There's no calorie difference and no healthiness gap, and cooking vegetables extends the range and variety of tastes and textures you can enjoy. Cooked vegetables seem more filling and satisfying, more like real food, especially if they're well-flavoured. How about grilled mushrooms, or stir-fried Chinese vegetables, or baked aubergine, or carrot and coriander soup, just for starters? These foods seem like real meals.

FLUID FACTS

Our bodies are filled with enough liquid to fill a good-sized puddle. If you've ever been stranded on sea or land without a drop to drink, you know how much you depend on a constant supply of fluids to keep you feeling hale and hearty.

But you don't have to be lost in the desert to suffer from dehydration. In general, you will lose 2 to 3 litres of water every day through breathing, perspiring, even sneezing. You lose more when the air is dry or stale — as in an aeroplane — or when the air is very hot or cold. Hence, the often-quoted recommendation that you should drink the equivalent of eight glasses of water every day.

But does it really have to be water? And how do you keep count? Here are some ways to measure your liquid assets without keeping a water meter running all the time.

Drink when you're thirsty. Some people believe they have to force themselves to drink those eight glasses of water if they're going to get enough liquids every day. Thirst is a fairly reliable indicator of the need for fluids. However, there are times when thirst may not be the best indicator — for example, when you're exercising strenuously.

Don't scorn fizzy or soft drinks. While pure water is the easiest, quickest, and probably the best way to get fluids into your body, you'd probably like to have a fizzy drink now and then. The fluid in these does count, especially if you're drinking a low-sodium, low-carbohydrate diet drink.

Gain from the garden. Fruit and vegetables definitely have fluids that contribute to your total daily consumption.

Count tea and coffee, too. It's a common misconception that the caffeine found in tea, coffee, or other caffeinated drinks actually 'drains' fluids from your system. Though caffeine is a mild diuretic, when you drink a caffeinated beverage, your body still retains as much as half the fluid.

What I'm saying, of course, is that I don't want you to think you have to eat the 'rabbit food' that many people associate with dieting. Cold, raw vegetables – lettuce leaves, sprouts, celery and carrot sticks – aren't for everyone. In fact, even people who love the rabbit-food veggies find there's only so much of them they can eat. So to the extent that cooked vegetables extend your vegetable options, they're a definite plus for weight loss.

Here's something I'm going to repeat a number of times throughout this book. If this advice becomes your mantra, so be it. It is simply this: eat as many vegetables as you want, any way you want them.

Use vegetables in soups and stews. Marinate them. Purée your vegetables, sauté them, chop them, pickle them, grill them, serve them with low-calorie sauces, dressings, relishes, chutneys, condiments, spices and herbs. It doesn't matter how you eat them, so long as you do eat them.

SALT AND WEIGHT LOSS

I would guess that about 95 per cent of my patients are concerned about their salt intake. Chronic dieters – and that includes a lot of the people who come to me – tend to assume that anything they like should be restricted, so they take it for granted that salty foods like soy sauce, pickles and soups are going to be bad for them.

But that's not necessarily so. Sodium, which plays a big role in the body's fluid balance, is not an issue when it comes to losing fat. There may be a medical reason for you to restrict your salt intake, but that's a matter to discuss with your medical doctor.

In fact, for two very obvious reasons, salt can actually help the weight-loss process. Firstly, salt has no calories. Secondly, salt

flavours food. All those sodium-packed dressings, sauces and condiments are flavoursome inducements to eat the vegetables, seafood and soups that make such good, low-calorie choices.

Your scales may well go up a pound or two if you choose such high-sodium foods as canned soup or tomato juice. But that's only because sodium tends to make you retain water. You really haven't gained or regained fat.

Similarly, if you eat a very low-salt diet for a while, especially if you're drinking a lot of fluid, you can trick your kidneys into dispelling a lot of water. You'll urinate a lot, so it may seem that you've lost weight. But you really haven't lost fat.

In both these situations, by the way, the normal balance will restore itself. As for fat loss, that will come, with or without salt, through calorie reduction and exercise.

DE GUSTIBUS

In matters of taste, the old saying goes, there's no point in arguing. In fact, differences in people's perception of flavours are rooted in their genes. So is your threshold of perception – as measured in the number of tastebuds you have.

Research has shown that about a quarter of us – the super-tasters – possess a higher number of tastebuds and experience flavours more intensely. Another quarter of us have fewer tastebuds than average. These people are known as non-tasters.

Super-tasters – who tend to be women, since oestrogen actually enhances taste perception – have a particular genetic sensitivity to a compound found in some vegetables, such as broccoli, that makes them feel strongly, one way or the other, about these foods. Non-tasters can be absolutely blind to this taste as well as to the so-called bitter aftertaste of such foods as artificial sweeteners.

THE SCALES ARE YOUR ENEMY

You walked to the office this morning and were on the move all day at work. You went to an exercise class after work. As soon as you got home, you stepped on the scales to see how well you'd done.

Sure enough, you lost 5 pounds! You're thrilled to have this knowledge before you head out to your favourite restaurant. This calls for a bit of a binge.

Think again. That easy 5-pound weight loss isn't really a fat loss after all. What you lost was water — all the sweat from that exercise at the gym. And because it was water your body needs, you will eventually get it back — along with the 'lost' 5 pounds on the scale.

Let's take another scenario, which might be just as likely to happen on another day. Again, you walked to the office and stayed on the move all day. Again, you put in your time at exercise class. Feeling confident about your weight loss for this day, you once again stepped on the scale as soon as you got home.

But . . . what's this?

Nothing lost! Not an ounce! The needle is right where it was this morning — maybe even a smidgen higher! All that effort for nothing. Might as well give up and binge!

Again, the scales have lied. What really happened is that you drank a lot today. Or maybe it was that salty soup you had for lunch. Or both. What's registering as a slight weight gain is a water gain — and it's as temporary as water loss.

The moral is this: let some time pass between weigh-ins. A stuck needle can be

A plateau in weight gain may be due to water, not calories

demoralising, especially when it may be due to water retention. If you can't stay away from looking at the scales, check your weight no more than once a week.

A better measure, if you want one, is to try on an article of clothing that either doesn't fit you at all or is very snug. Then, try it on again once every 10 days to see how it fits you differently. The clothing doesn't change size, so any difference in the way it fits is an indication that you're losing weight.

THAT BEDTIME SNACK

It's a Spanish tradition: have your last meal late at night, not long before you head for bed.

Eating right before bedtime? Isn't that an invitation to obesity?

Evidently not. There's now scientific evidence that you don't gain more weight if you eat late at night. Several studies confirm that when you eat has no connection with weight, and that evening eating has no more effect on your weight than morning eating. It's the total number of calories consumed daily and expended in activity that makes — or breaks — weight gain.

Apparently, the time of day when you consume those calories or burn them is really not an issue. The calories in your bedtime snack will be burned when they're needed. Even sleep burns about 50 calories an hour.

NO TIME FORBIDDEN

'Eat your main meal at lunch, not dinner… Eat a healthy breakfast, whether you're hungry or not… Eat several small meals throughout the day, rather than three meals at specific times… Eat three meals a day at regular intervals and at the same time each day… Eat nothing after 9 p.m.' Does any of this sound familiar?

We're deluged with helpful hints, tips, prescriptions, schedules, instructions and formulas about when to eat and when not to eat. Here's my advice: forget it all.

Don't check the clock to see when to eat. Eat when you're hungry. Your body will tell you when it needs food. And while there may be some small benefit to be gained in terms of energy or weight loss or overall health from each of the decrees listed above, what really counts is the number of calories you consume in a 24-hour period.

I see no particular advantage in eating a big breakfast – or any breakfast at all – if you're not hungry. And if you are hungry and want to eat at 4 a.m., be my guest. At any time of day or night, food *choices*, not timing, will be the factor that makes the biggest difference to your weight.

PLAYING THE NUMBERS

'How many calories should I eat in order to lose weight?' It's the question everyone asks and no one can answer. I can't either. I won't give patients a specific number, and I certainly can't come up with a number for the readers of this book.

But this much I can promise: if you take in fewer calories than you need to maintain your present weight, you will lose pounds. That's why this book focuses on expanding your awareness. Once you know there are low-calorie alternatives to what you're

currently eating, you free yourself from the calorie-counting competition.

Needless to say, if you're curious about the calories in a specific food, it's easy to determine that. Just check the nutrition label on the packet. Comparable foods often do have slightly different calorie counts.

But, frankly, a few calories one way or another, a few more calories one day than another, make little difference and are beside the point. The real goal is finding a way to eat that is comfortable for you – and a way of eating that you can continue over a lifetime. The point is to change your relationship with food in a positive way.

A SMALL-PORTION SOLUTION

Most of my patients instinctively assume that they are eating too much. They're pretty sure that if they could just cut their portions in half, they would lose weight.

But if you need X amount of food to feel satisfied, which is what you're eating now, half of X simply will not work. You'll end up

> **To feel good, you need to fulfil your cravings**

feeling deprived, which inevitably will lead you to the place you don't want to be. Deprivation, in fact, is the enemy of the person trying to lose weight. It's a set-up for regaining the weight you lose.

To me, portion cutting seems like an ill-advised exercise in a false kind of willpower. And it's not necessary. The truth is that most weight-conscious people aren't eating enough. What they really need is larger quantities of lower-calorie food. They need to eat enough to satisfy both their senses and their psyches.

SABOTEUR FOODS

'Saboteur foods' are foods that pretend to help you lose weight. But the fact is, these foods serve no purpose in weight control. They are the high-calorie/empty-calorie foods that we give ourselves permission to eat because they are lower in fat or sugar than their 'normal' food counterparts.

All too typically, when we give ourselves permission to eat these foods, we can easily rationalise overeating them. That is why saboteur foods are the only foods I suggest you avoid in my weight-loss programme. Quite simply, they will sabotage your weight-loss efforts and undermine the results.

High on the list of saboteurs are low-fat and fat-free baked goods. To read the advertising on these products, you'd think weight would vanish in an instant. The evidence – and there's lots of it – shows otherwise. All you're really doing is exchanging one kind of calorie for another.

There are many other saboteurs besides these obviously misleading (and oh so tempting) baked goods. In fact, I divide saboteur foods into two main categories: the have-nots, and the haves.

The have-nots are all those snack foods with advertising that lists all the 'bad' ingredients they do not contain. They are low-fat, reduced-fat, sugar-free, low-sodium and so on. The no-cholesterol claim is the one that really gets my goat. Cholesterol-free foods can still be high in ingredients that really add weight. Crisps and chips, for example, have no cholesterol, but they are loaded with fats and are very high in calories.

The other category of saboteur foods – the ones I call haves – are the ones I refer to as 'healthy naturals'. We mistakenly perceive these foods as having some redeeming nutritional benefit.

REDUCED TO WHAT?

If you're a cheese lover who's also watching your weight by shopping for reduced-fat cheese, here's an eye-opener: a 50g chunk of reduced-fat cheese has as much fat and as many calories as a 50g chunk of salami. In fact, many reduced-fat cheeses have the same number of calories as the richest Brie or Camembert in the cheese shop. So ... which would you rather eat?

Our staff nutritionist says she has seen more people gain weight on fat-free biscuits than on any other food. It's easy to rationalise that they're both healthy and low-calorie, especially if it takes half the packet to make you feel full. But consider this: a whole melon has the same calorie count as a single fat-free biscuit. And not only that: the melon also has a generous helping of fibre, vitamins and minerals.

Carob is a classic food saboteur. It seems nutritionally correct and bills itself as the low-fat answer to chocolate. But, in fact, it is a substitute that has the same fat and calorie content as real chocolate — thanks to the processing that turned the carob into a snack bar. If it's chocolate you want, eat chocolate.

Maybe the product is sweetened with fruit juice or honey instead of with refined sugar. Or the snack bar is made of carob instead of chocolate. Perhaps the crisps are made from vegetables other than potatoes. The list goes on and on. The replacement item sounds healthy and natural, so we rationalise that it isn't as bad as an empty-calorie food.

But a biscuit sweetened with honey is just as high in calories as one sweetened with sugar. And crisps made from sweet potatoes or parsnips, instead of from regular white spuds, differ from traditional potato crisps only in content, not in calories. They're not any better for you.

BEING CAUGHT OUT

Most of the time, you're better off eating 'real' biscuits or crisps rather than one of the 'have-not' or 'have' saboteur alternatives.

Here's why. Even if a saboteur is lower in fat, sugar or calories than the regular food, it's almost certain you'll give yourself permission to eat them more frequently – and probably in more generous quantities. Over time, then, they'll add more calories.

It's easy to find out whether these foods are high in calories. Just check the nutritional information on the label. But it's unlikely you'll do that. Instead, we tend to rationalise by saying, 'Well, I really need to have a biscuit – and since I'm going to have a biscuit anyway, it might as well be low-fat.' In other words, it's easy to fall into the habit of thinking the so-called diet biscuit is 'not as bad'.

But look what happens. Since the diet biscuit isn't nearly as good as the one it's replacing, you eat more in an effort to satisfy yourself. See why I dub these foods saboteurs?

Certainly, not all low-fat or sugar-free foods are useless. As you'll see in the pages that follow, I recommend many and include them on the Anytime List of foods on page 138. And as the visual demonstrations throughout the book make clear, there is a range of low-calorie foods you can eat in any quantity whenever you like. But beware the food saboteurs!

THE OLESTRA STORY

With the Western world clamouring for low-fat foods, researchers at food companies have been hard-pressed to come up with substitutes. And the one substitute that seems to fit the bill has been the source of a lot of controversy.

Synthetically produced olestra is a fat substitute that is not absorbed by the digestive system. Common in the USA, it is occasionally found in savoury snacks, such as crisps, elsewhere. Not only is it calorie-free, it is also free of cholesterol and can be used in deep frying. Best of all, it tastes good. What a bonanza: olestra potato crisps that taste like the real thing and have fewer calories than baked or fat-free crisps. Too good to be true?

It just may be, because there's a painful downside to olestra. In many people, anything more than a very small amount of olestra-filled food may cause harsh stomach cramps and diarrhoea. What's more, researchers still have not determined how olestra may affect the body's absorption of the fat-soluble vitamins A, E, D and K. Though the manufacturers have enriched their olestra products with additional amounts of these vitamins, they may leave the body along with the unabsorbed fat.

This means that eating large quantities of the good-tasting, reduced-calorie olestra foods may deplete your supply of fat-soluble vitamins. You may also lose carotenoids – like beta-carotene – that function as antioxidants and play a role in preventing diseases, such as cancer and heart disease. We just can't say for certain how much of these nutrients you're losing and what the long-term effects are. Until we know more, I'd recommend small quantities of olestra at infrequent intervals. Even better, have none at all.

CRAVING AND APPETITE: IS IT ALL IN YOUR HEAD?

We think of appetite as a generalised desire for something – for sweets, perhaps, or for 'something salty'. And we think of a craving as an extreme, almost obsessive requirement for a specific food – as when you absolutely have to have a hot fudge sundae.

> **Cravings are born out of a number of complex factors**

The truth is that there is no known mechanism in the human body that translates a physiological need for a nutrient into a yearning for a food that is high in that nutrient. What's more, as everybody knows, the cravings that attack us are rarely for foods that are good for us. When was the last time you felt you just 'had to have' a plate of broccoli? But how about a rich chocolate brownie? You can probably work up a good craving for that without too much trouble.

Cravings come from an interaction of neurochemical, nutritional, cultural and psychological factors, all working together in ways we don't clearly understand. But that doesn't mean they're not real. They're very real – and quite powerful.

Searching for the mechanism that helps control appetite, researchers at the University of California at Irvine College of Medicine have discovered a receptor in the brain that is a major regulator of eating. The receptor binds to a nervous system chemical called melanin-concentrating hormone (MCH), which is known to regulate how often and how much we eat. A drug that blocks the receptor would probably control overeating, but experts don't expect such a drug to be available for at least 10 years.

DEPRIVATION AND CRAVINGS

One hint about how appetite works is that a craving is usually for something we consider tasty and satisfying but that we don't allow ourselves to eat on a regular basis. Chronic dieters are seized by cravings much more frequently than non-dieters. That's because food deprivation and/or loss of body fat can have a profound influence on the same brain chemicals that regulate appetite. The maddeningly skinny person who never diets isn't deprived; she might want ice cream from time to time but won't obsess about it. But the dieter will change her mind 15 times about the flavour, endlessly debate about the topping and worry about the consequences of going off her diet.

PLANNED BINGEING

The next time you feel a craving coming on, ask yourself what you really want. Is it the hot fudge sundae? Will a frozen yoghurt do just as well? A craving can often be satisfied by a lower-calorie food of similar flavour or texture. But sometimes, you just have to go for the sundae.

I know that 'planned bingeing' sounds like a contradiction in terms. After all,

HORMONES AND TASTE

One factor that appears to work with the 'appetite chemicals' are hormones. Women are known to have more cravings than men.

Everybody knows that pregnant women are often seized by sudden tastes for salty or spicy food. The same thing happens premenstrually. Changing hormone levels affect the taste perception of salt, raising the salt taste threshold. Saltier, more savoury, more highly flavoured foods seem more appealing to women during these times.

bingeing implies something done impulsively, in an out-of-control way. The image that comes to mind is of eating a whole packet of biscuits at one sitting, or scoffing down a huge bag of crisps. It's something done hurriedly, almost furtively, as if consuming a large quantity of high-calorie food were an evil deed.

By planning your binge, however – by preceding it with thought and executing it in the context of a decision – you can get all the enjoyment you deserve without remorse.

Consider one of my successful patients, Annie. Annie had always found that dipping into the bread basket would trigger an eating binge that would make her unhappy afterwards. After a minimal amount of Food Awareness Training, she came in to report a wonderful experience of the day before:

'I met a friend for lunch and had a delicious meal of fish and grilled vegetables. On the way home, I passed my favourite Italian bakery. They were just putting out some freshly baked bread, and the smell was overwhelming. I went inside and bought a sesame-seed loaf. In the past, I would have eaten a few pieces and felt completely out of control. But this time, I enjoyed every bite of it, and I didn't feel guilty.'

You can gain enjoyment without gaining weight

The bread had 840 calories, and it certainly wasn't a nutritionally adequate meal. But since Annie had eaten low-calorie, healthy food during the rest of the day, her personal bread binge didn't produce either weight gain, nutritional deficiency or guilt. As Annie herself said, she felt good about herself. Rather than making the mistake of eating

something that didn't really satisfy her urge, Annie had enjoyed her binge, right down to the last, delicious morsel.

Whatever your binge trigger is – bread or chocolate or crisps, even cassoulet – when you make the decision to eat it, enjoy it.

BOREDOM

Food is not boring. Diets are. One reason diets never work is that people simply tire of eating the same food over and over again. It's a great incentive to 'cheat'. That won't happen

If you have a broad range of choices, you won't get bored

on the picture perfect weight-loss programme because no food is ruled out. You're not restricted to eating certain foods in certain quantities. Quite the contrary – I want to broaden the scope of your food choices.

NO FAILURE IMPLIED

When someone lets their diet lapse, they typically express the retreat as a failure. There's a moral undertone to it all: they've had a 'bad day'. A character flaw is implied. Feelings of self-worth can plummet; confidence takes a dive; the whole weight-loss effort suffers.

Patients usually adapt to my weight-loss programme very quickly, not just because they're motivated but also because the choices offered are very easy to live with. But many of my patients have days in which they don't lose weight. That's natural. It's human. It says nothing about your moral character. Expect it. Recognise that you will have some days when you consume more calories than other days, and keep moving on. This is a process, and that what you are doing is changing your relationship with food.

STARTING THE PICTURE PERFECT PROGRAMME

A journey of a thousand miles must begin with a single step, the saying goes.

That's the way to think of the weight-loss programme in this book, too – not as a diet but as a first step on a journey into awareness that will continue forever, your opening stride into a life-changing experience.

For the most part, new patients making first-time appointments with me are referred to my office by other patients who are happy with their success. But I have one patient in particular who operates with an especially missionary-like zeal.

Her name is Karen. When a new patient is referred to me by Karen, I never know where they may have met. She may have had a conversation with a customer under the next hair dryer at the hairdresser's. Or she may have been speaking to a fellow guest at a wedding. Or she just started talking to the chap sitting beside her on the train. I don't know how these conversations get started, but as soon as the topic of weight comes up, pretty soon she has convinced whoever she's talking to that he or she should get involved with my programme.

One day about a year ago, Karen turned up at my office unannounced at midday. She had been lunching with a good friend and had managed to bring him directly to my office from the restaurant.

Definitely a first. Most people don't want to meet a weight-control expert straight after a slap-up lunch. Karen's friend was good-natured and gentlemanly about being 'kidnapped', however, and I tried to allay what I was certain was his reluctance. I told him he didn't have to start the programme because Karen was talking him into it. I explained the programme and sent him home to think about it before he made a decision.

Today's the day to start changing what you eat

I wasn't sure when or if I'd hear from him, but 5 days later, he called. Now, 6 months later, he has lost 3½ stone and he can't thank me enough. I tell him it's not me he should thank, it's Karen. The truth is that thanks are owed to whatever internal force said to him, 'Okay, today's the day'.

WHAT BRINGS YOU HERE?

In a study of people who had lost at least 2 stone and had kept the weight off for at least a year, every one of those people said they could identify a particular 'moment of truth' – a specific triggering incident or realisation – that helped them get started on weight loss.

For one patient of mine, it was an inspiring article in a magazine. For another, it was seeing herself in a full-length mirror. Someone told me he couldn't play with his son without wheezing. Another person was walking down the street and caught sight of her own reflection in a department store window.

Some come to see me because they have been advised by their doctors to lose weight for medical reasons – perhaps the threat of diabetes, evidence of high blood pressure or maybe a high cholesterol count. Other patients have been thin all their lives but are experiencing middle-aged spread.

Others have put weight on in the wake of a traumatic experience – perhaps the end of a marriage or love affair, or maybe a professional crisis or anxieties associated with the onset of middle age.

Sometimes people tell me they've carried around an article about my programme for 2 years, and now here they are. I tell them how glad I am that they rushed into it.

POWER IN UNDERSTANDING

While every patient coming into my office has his or her own reason for being there, all share a similar need to change their relationship with food. The way we get them started on that change is not with a weigh-in. Once someone has made that all-important first move through the door of the office, he or she has an initial consultation with me, with my staff nutritionist, and with a staff psychologist. That's because all three disciplines – the medical, the nutritional and the psychological – come into play in understanding the nature of each person's relationship with food.

If someone is going to be empowered to change that relationship, all three influences need to be considered. The change will show up on the scales. But that's not where the process of change begins – nor where it ends.

One thing I've come to understand over the years is that each person has an individual pattern in his or her relationship with food. I've seen those patterns emerge time and again over the years in the thousands of people we've helped. Whatever the individual's dieting history, whatever the trigger that has propelled the person into my office, these patterns are most profoundly influenced by lifestyle.

Clarifying your eating profile is essential for change

In fact, just about everybody falls into one of four eating 'profiles', which include not only a particular lifestyle but also the eating habits that go along with it. Before people begin to make changes, they need to recognise their eating habits.

THE FOUR CLASSIC PROFILES

The profiles are so real that I've named them after actual patients who best exemplified their classic characteristics:

- Susan was the classic example of the office worker tied to a desk.
- There's the business traveller, wined and dined round the clock – that was Stan.
- The mother at home all day with with young children was Diana – to a T.
- The student or shift worker who always eats on the run is personified by Doug.

After the initial consultation, I ask people to keep a food diary, recording as accurately as possible what they are eating, the situation and time in which they are eating and the degree of hunger they feel at the time. On the following pages you'll find the food diaries of Susan, Stan, Diana and Doug before they started my weight-loss programme. These diaries exemplify perfectly the four classic eating profiles. Now, I realise you might not be an office worker, a business executive, a mother with young children or a student or shift worker. But I'm willing to bet my practice that you'll recognise your own eating profile in one of these four scenarios.

EATING PROFILE NUMBER 1: TIED-TO-A-DESK

Susan once told me that she believes she has thought about food for 45 of every 60 seconds of her life. Despite being on a diet 'half the time', she always believes she's the fattest person in the room 'and the only one who's starving'. These words could serve as a slogan for the classic eating profile embodied by the tied-to-a-desk office worker.

The rhythm of the day is tied to food and thoughts of food

Sound familiar? Chances are, you start every day with the conscious vow not to eat. You're filled with resolve – alert, alive, purposeful. You take your place in the queue at the sandwich counter, cafeteria or tea trolley, determined to have only coffee this morning. But somehow, you hear yourself asking for the danish pastry as well.

'Sometimes,' says Susan, 'I buy the diet doughnut instead – plain, no sugar, no jam. That has to be a few calories less, doesn't it?'

Stress makes you eat, and worry leads to stress, and I'll bet that one of the things that worries you most is being overweight. Maybe, as with Susan, there's a family history of heart disease or diabetes or some other condition – and you know that weight loss could literally save your life. 'But that doesn't seem to scare me enough into doing something about it,' says Susan.

Anyway, most of us can find some way to avoid taking action. Susan stopped running because of a bad knee. And because she's an accountant, she's unbelievably busy and pressured from January to April, so she says she 'really can't get anything going during those months'. But that comment makes her pause. 'Not that the rest of the year is easy,' she finally adds.

You probably eat lunch at your desk. And I wouldn't be surprised if you usually order from the same old place – and, often, order the same lunch you had yesterday and the day before that.

Or maybe you head for the company cafeteria. There, you try to keep it light. Susan's usual meal is 'a chicken Caesar salad or, if I'm truly cutting back, salad and chicken with just an oil and vinegar dressing and maybe a bread stick or two. Sometimes if I really, really want dessert, I get rice pudding.'

Your work is hard – nobody says otherwise – and by late afternoon, your energy is flagging. Someone in the office always keeps sweets or nuts on her desk. You certainly would never keep a supply on your own desk – you're too afraid your mouth would be full all the time – but you do occasionally dip into

It is easy to be tempted by office vending machines

their bowl. And I wouldn't be surprised if you buy a replacement supply in bulk for that colleague every now and then, just so you don't feel too uncomfortable about helping yourself from time to time.

Susan will go to the vending machine if she wants a snack. She gets the low-fat biscuits or a low-fat cereal bar, which she thinks is better than a chocolate bar.

When work is over, she and a crowd of colleagues go out for a drink. The bar serves snacks during its happy hour. Susan tries to resist, but then goes for the chicken wings and meatballs. These seem to her to be the best choice. They're protein, at least.

SUSAN'S FOOD DIARY

Time	Food	Hunger level (0–4)	Situation	Comments
9.00am	Dry bagel and unsweetened grapefruit juice	3	Working at desk	Starting good day of dieting
Noon	White-meat turkey on rye-bread with mustard	3	Working at desk	Still on diet
3.00pm	Reduced-fat biscuits (one packet)	3	Coffee break at vending machine	Feeling low; need an energy booster
6.30pm	Chinese takeaway: steamed veg with beef, Plain rice, ½ spring roll	3	Watching TV at home	Tasteless diet meal; ate half a spring roll, threw half away; had to have it
9.00pm	Low-fat ice cream (¼ container). One slice low-fat cake, frozen	1	Talking on phone in kitchen	Wanted something sweet but didn't go out of control. Not a bad diet day

Then it's off home. You've had a long, hard day, some nibbles you could have done without and a drink or two. The fact is, you're really hungry. Susan says she usually has a couple of glasses of juice to take the edge off her appetite. 'Then, if I'm feeling up to it, I'll make myself a grilled chicken breast. But then I'm still hungry. I'll have a bag of carrot sticks, but it's like eating medicine.'

After medicine, of course, you deserve to have something you really want. Susan might have low-fat cheese and biscuits. Then, after the salty stuff, she wants something sweet. So she has some low-fat ice cream or a reduced-fat cake from the freezer and she tucks into that. She doesn't care if it's frozen.

When you look back over Susan's day, it has been virtually defined by food. Does this ring a bell?

MY NOTES ON SUSAN:

Susan consumes fruit juice – a bad calorie buy – in the mistaken view that it's low in sugar and calories. In fact, it's loaded with both.

She eats tasteless, bland 'diet food' all day and doubtless consumes far more calories than she realises. She's constantly hungry, too. I suggest more filling, tasty alternatives. Susan could be eating a larger quantity of enjoyable food for far fewer calories. She has a very low intake of fibre-rich fruits and vegetables.

Analysis: Susan is the typical 'dieter'. She goes for the low-fat choice in the mistaken assumption that it's the solution to her weight problem. She is unaware that low-fat does not necessarily mean low-calorie. Moreover, her food choices are so boring that she needs the high-fat, high-calorie spring roll at dinner as compensation for the persistent tastelessness of her eating.

EATING PROFILE NUMBER 2: BUSINESS TRAVELLER

Stan doesn't quite grasp the concept of moderation. Sound familiar? Well, if you're the type of person who works hard and plays hard, you probably eat whenever, wherever and whatever is necessary for fuel.

To a person who travels a lot on business, eating is often an integral part of work. A lot of your most important meetings and conferences take place at mealtimes. The power breakfast, the working lunch, the dinner with customers: these are at the core of your professional life. You're expected to partake. But certain parts of this equation – like when, where or what you eat – are not in

> ## You may not know where or when you'll be eating next

your control. Consider overseas travel. Juggling time zones and coping with jet lag is no picnic. Did you sleep on the plane? If not, your body is confused about whether or not it's a meal time.

Nothing's certain about the next meal, either. If you travel by plane, you can never really be sure what they'll be serving for the onboard meal or snack – if anything. That's why a lot of business travellers eat on a kind of contingency basis. Stan finds he often eats in preparation for the possibility of not finding time to eat later. He'll pick up a muffin and coffee to eat in the car en route to the office, where he tries to squeeze in at least an hour of work before leaving on a business trip.

Later, at the airport, 'I'll grab a roll or something because I'm not sure what they will be serving on the plane. Or else I'll just wait, hope they serve something and eat whatever they serve.'

Eat what's available when it's available: that seems to be the mantra. If you're the typical business traveller, you no doubt feel you're at the mercy of a schedule set by others. And you want to be at your best at all times. That's why you need the fuel that food provides, and why you worry about exactly when you'll get the next chance to fill up – and on what.

A weight-loss diet for someone like Stan? Forget about it. 'I can't plan ahead when I'm on the road. I'm not in charge. I've tried following diets, but believe me, you can't carry your meals around in your briefcase or tell your colleagues that you can have only 150 grams of lamb for dinner. It just doesn't work.'

Conferences, seminars and executive briefings are especially challenging. They're always putting food in front of you. At lunch, says Stan, 'they just set out sandwiches and biscuits, and I have no choice. The same with dinner at a conference: it's a set menu. Nothing I can do about it.'

Or maybe you're staying in a hotel. There's the hotel dining room, of course, but if you've arrived late, you're probaby looking forward to tucking into something in the quiet of your room. But 'the choices in room service tend to be really limited,' Stan says. Your alternative to room service? A chocolate bar and a bag of peanuts from the mini bar.

At last the day or week of travel is finished. By the time you do get home, Stan complains, 'it's too late to get a normal dinner since it's way past everyone else's dinnertime, so I scavenge whatever I can find in the cupboard or fridge.'

Even at home at the weekend, the busy executive is frequently either entertaining or being entertained. Dinner out ritually begins with a drink or two. For Stan, 'if I make the mistake of having a second drink, my guard goes down and I'm not very careful about what I'm ordering for dinner. I always just think I'll go to the gym – tomorrow.'

MY NOTES ON STAN

Stan eats in the car. Nothing wrong with this – there's no wrong place or time to eat. But he can find a lower calorie alternative to the muffin that is equally convenient and satisfying.

Stan is sometimes eating for social reasons when he isn't hungry. He can still sit down and eat in such situations, but when he is aware of what he is doing, he may be able to make better choices. He should become aware of lower-calorie choices that are available – and that he would enjoy – in the types of restaurants in which he is dining. At the moment, he consumes several high-calorie, high-fat foods at the same meal.

Stan experiences his most severe hunger at dinnertime. I suggest having a start-off food – soup or a starter – to take the edge off his appetite early in the meal.

I also suggest ordering a sparkling mineral water instead of the first alcoholic drink. Stan should alternate glasses of water and wine to cut wine consumption. Note that he probably would not have consumed the chocolate bar if alcohol at dinner hadn't lowered his resistance.

A good rule of thumb: never insert the key into the mini bar. There's nothing in there that is a good calorie choice.

Analysis: Stan's business and professional life is not going to change. But these circumstances won't be difficult to deal with when he is more informed about eating, calories and nutrition.

STAN'S FOOD DIARY

Time	Food	Hunger level (0–4)	Situation	Comments
8.00am	Bran muffin (150g)	2	Driving to work	On way to a presentation
9.00am	2 scrambled eggs, 3 rashers bacon, hashbrown potatoes, bagel with butter	1	Restaurant breakfast meeting	Not very hungry
1.00pm	Chicken caesar salad. Few bread sticks	2	Talking in restaurant	Business lunch
8.00pm	Scotch. Mozzarella penne a la vodka. Roll and butter, 2 glasses of wine	4	Business dinner in restaurant	
11.00pm	Large chocolate bar from mini bar	2	Watching TV in hotel room	Not really hungry, want something sweet

EATING PROFILE NUMBER 3: MOTHER AT HOME

Diana – the person who best fits the home-with-the-kids profile – rarely sits down to a meal, but she weighs more today than she ever has, and she can't quite figure out why.

How can you gain weight when you only eat some scraps here, a few bites of this, some morsels of leftovers – what does it all add up to? Well, snacking can add up to a lot if you do it all day long.

First thing in the morning, Diana makes breakfast for the kids. As she's pouring cereal into each bowl, she pops a few handfuls of flakes into her mouth. The kids eat, she gets them packed up, sees them off on the school bus – the usual hectic morning in a family with young children. She comes home to a quiet house and a messy kitchen and polishes off the uneaten cereal left behind.

Her day has begun. Diana cuts a tiny slice of the coffee cake she bought for her husband, Joe, and nibbles at it as she picks up some of the kids' toys. When she does the laundry, she helps herself to another slice of cake. A neighbour drops by. Diana takes a break from

DIANA'S FOOD DIARY

Time	Food	Hunger level (0–4)	Situation	Comments
8.00am	Few handfuls of low-fat muesli	0	Kitchen, feeding kids	Busy
8.45am	Small slice coffee cake	1	Kitchen, folding laundry	Cake bought for husband
10.00am	Handful of cheese crackers	0	On way to get vacuum	Grabbed handful from box on counter
1.00pm	Green salad with oil and vinegar. 4 crackers. Muffin, dry	3	With friends in restaurant	In the 'who-can-eat-less' competition; ordered muffin as better choice than cake
3.00pm	Choc ice	0	At ice-cream van with kids after school	Not really hungry, want something sweet
6.00pm	Left over macaroni and cheese (small bowl)	3	Nibbled kids' leftovers	
8.00pm	¼ roast chicken (170g) with rice and vegetables	1	Dining room with husband	
10.00pm	3 chocolate-chip cookies	1	Preparing kids' lunch boxes	Exhausted

housework and brews some coffee. When the neighbour accepts Diana's offer of a slice of cake, Diana also cuts a sliver for herself.

Without a job to go to anymore, Diana helps out at her children's school. She likes the companionship. For the volunteers there are tea and biscuits. Taking some biscuits from the edge of the plate, Diana instinctively rearranges the rest, so no one notices any have been taken. In fact, people are constantly commenting that she hardly eats a thing, even though Diana knows that they're wondering why, then, she isn't thinner.

Diana used to have a full-time job outside the home – and when she did, she was a lot thinner. 'Weight was never a problem,' she recalls. She assumes she'll go back to work when the kids are grown up, and she certainly hopes the weight loss will be 'automatic' then. But, rationally, that's beginning to seem more and more unlikely.

After the birth of her first baby, Diana gained 3 stone. She lost most of that weight, but then came the second baby and more pounds. When she first came to see me, Diana was 4 stone over her wedding-dress weight. 'I used to be able to do handstands. Now I can barely run around after the kids all day. I'm not that old, but I don't have any energy.'

She tries to eat foods that are 'not so bad', as she puts it. At lunch with a friend shortly before she first came to see me, she ordered tuna salad, no bread. But the tuna salad came with potato salad. It wasn't her fault. She didn't ask for it. But she ate it anyway.

For dessert, she ordered a plain muffin. It was a boring choice – so she reckoned it couldn't be too fattening. She really wanted the chocolate cake but didn't allow herself.

Daily life for Diana is driven by her children's needs. It's a fact of life, but it also influences her eating. When she picks the children up from school and takes them for a treat, she has one too. It's a time of day when she's tired anyway, so an ice cream serves as an energy-booster.

Diana's day is punctuated by unconscious snacking

In the evening, she usually cooks two dinners – one for the kids and a second meal for Joe. She'll pick at what the kids are eating, then snack on wheat crackers or bread sticks because she gets hungry waiting for Joe. She eats a little something with him because he doesn't like to eat alone. 'Joe isn't really a help. He'll say, "Do you really want that?" and I'll say, "Yes, I do," and I'll eat it even if I don't really want it. If you asked him, he'd say he's being supportive.'

There's generally nothing for dessert. (What happened to that coffee cake anyway?) So sometimes, late at night, Diana will munch on the kids' peanut butter on crackers.

MY NOTES ON DIANA

Diana nibbles all day long and never sits down to a real meal. She is completely out of touch with whether she is really hungry or not and needs focus. She is taking in a tremendous number of calories. She also has a few misconceptions, such as thinking that a plain muffin has fewer calories than the cake she really wants.

If Diana's lifestyle really requires eating little bits of food all day, there are better foods she can keep on hand, such as boiled sweets, fruit and low-calorie ice lollies.

Analysis: classic mindless eating. Diana is simply not paying attention. She is not focused on the fact that she is eating, not to mention on the choices she is making.

EATING PROFILE NUMBER 4: STUDENT OR SHIFT-WORKER

Maybe it started when you were at university – and doing part-time work as well. Your commitments kept you busy. When other people were sitting down to lunch or dinner, you were studying, working or some combination of both. Or maybe it's the nature of your job. When normal mealtimes come around, your working day is just getting under way. Either you don't feel like eating, or you can't take a break right then.

Whatever the cause, the reality is that you eat on the run – when you can and where you can. On a non-schedule like this, whatever you see is probably going to be what you eat.

Doug is a police officer. When he first came into my office, he certainly looked the part of the *Mean Streets* cop – big, burly, with a lot more in the midsection than he wanted to be there.

Doug says he was always generously proportioned. By the time he got to college, however, he was 'constantly snacking'. Back then, he says, 'I had a well-established beer-and-chips habit.'

> ## 'You don't get the cool clothes in my size'

Today, Doug concedes he feels a certain amount of embarrassment about his kind of bulk. 'When it comes to wearing great clothes and meeting new people, I'd rather be slim,' he says. 'Most women seem to go more for a Brad Pitt kind of man. It's a self-esteem issue.'

But what's a police officer to do if he works difficult hours like the noon-to-eight shift? He's working while others are having lunch and dinner, and he's sleeping while the rest of the world has breakfast.

Since Doug sleeps till 10 or 11 a.m., he just skips breakfast. He usually goes out to lunch at 2 or 3 p.m., 'because I'm really hungry by then. So I'll have something like a burger and fries, or steak and eggs and chips, anything that comes along. Anyway, it's two meals in one – lunch and the breakfast I didn't have earlier.'

Without a regular, 'normal' schedule of meals to sit down to, dinner is often a takeaway. 'What usually happens is that someone will yell out, "Does anyone want anything from the café?" and I'll look at the clock and it's 7 or 8 p.m., so I'll yell back, "Yeah, get me whatever you're having", and that'll be pie and mash or whatever the special is.'

For variation? 'Maybe a few of us will go out to eat. We tend to look for a place that will give us the most food for the least money. It's kind of crazy – we'll go where the portions are biggest even if the food isn't that good. We just want more on the plate. We like the kind of places that give you soup, salad, bread, the main meal and dessert. That's what I had yesterday, at an Italian place.' Then the shift ends, and what could be more natural than a couple of drinks with the lads – especially at the end of a stressful day?

On the way home, Doug says, he'll usually stop at a McDonald's, especially if he hasn't eaten anything in a few hours. 'It's a meal, I guess, but to me it's a snack: a big Mac, large fries and a Coke and oh, yeah, why don't you throw in an apple pie while you're at it? I'll eat it all in the car.'

The quantities may seem unusual, but the pattern is not. There are many, many people these days with unconventional schedules. And that means unconventional eating habits.

DOUG'S FOOD DIARY				
Time	Food	Hunger level (0–4)	Situation	Comments
10.00am	McDonald's sausage and egg muffin	2	Reading paper in restaurant	Not really hungry
2.00pm	2 slices pepperoni pizza with coke	3	Lunchtime	Pizza was what everyone ordered
6.30pm	2 pieces of garlic bread, spaghetti bolognese, caesar salad, apple danish, cappuccino	3	Eating with a friend in restaurant	Big portions
11.00pm	Cheeseburger, fries and coke	1	In car	Feeling stuffed

Eventually, of course, this kind of eating will catch up with you. When Doug came to see me, he'd been through a fairly typical crash-diet experience. On a pre-packaged plan, Doug had lost a lot of weight fast. Then the plan faded into the background, old habits took over, and Doug put the weight back on just as quickly – and a little extra.

Doug grabs whatever tastes good, hungry or not

Determinedly, he tried again. 'I went to Weight Watchers and kept the weight off for a year and a half. Then all of a sudden I wasn't paying any attention, and because I had lost the weight, I was saying, "Oh well, I'm not fat anymore, I can eat anything. I don't have to pay attention." That's how I eat a lot of the time,' he concedes. 'There isn't a lot of planning. I just grab what I can and don't think much about it.'

MY NOTES ON DOUG

Doug eats when he's not hungry. He eats to be one of the gang, part of the crowd. There's no focus to his choices. He allows his odd working schedule to be the excuse for eating as a social event.

Doug needs to be more assertive about the restaurants he goes to as much as he needs to be more knowledgeable about food choices. His crowd prizes quantity over quality. Quantity is not necessarily a problem, but Doug could eat the same quantity if his choices were better.

Analysis: Doug needs basic nutrition education and more focus. Put the two together and he could be making healthy, low-calorie food choices despite the odd routine of his eating, the group choices of restaurant and his desire for large quantities.

WHAT'S YOUR PROFILE?

I don't think any of us fits exactly into one category. These are individuals – and each of us has individual lifestyle challenges to deal with. But I think it's important to recognise and respect the power of a lifestyle to influence our eating habits. Whether you're tied to an office job or you travel a lot on business, whether you're at home with the kids or working unorthodox hours, it's both impossible and unnecessary to completely change your lifestyle just because you want to lose weight.

But if your lifestyle won't change, what can? This is where these profiles are useful. All four of these individuals were able to get results with Food Awareness Training. Some lost more; some less. But all of them found a way to eat well, satisfy their appetites, keep their responsibilities going (just as before!) and, at the same time, develop the eating habits that enabled them to keep the weight off.

The truth is that all the people I've profiled were eating for different reasons but in the same way. They ate thoughtlessly – if not mindlessly. They really weren't paying attention to their eating or thinking about their food. That's why they were not really *choosing* what they ate. Instead, they let the situation, their emotions, or somebody else's schedule choose for them.

THE FOOD DIARY

Of course, there are lots of ways you can make low-calorie choices without keeping a diary. But if you really want the benefits that come with Food Awareness Training, keeping a diary – even for a short time – is absolutely the most helpful thing you can do for yourself. The food diary will help you evaluate your own food choices and eating behaviour, just as it helps my team of weight-loss experts analyse the food choices

and eating behaviour of my patients. As I well know, however, the mere thought of a food diary can provoke all sorts of negative reactions. One reaction is fear: do I really want anyone to know what it's like to be me, eating the food that I eat?

You'll learn to be in touch with how you feel about food

Then there's another reaction – well, let's call it a tendency to stretch the truth a little bit. It's a lot easier to say, 'I had a few snacks yesterday' than to recall and write down every snack you ate at different times of the day.

Plus, I can see how you might resist the requirement of having your diary handy and your pen ready through the day. Who wants to be bothered with writing this stuff down, meal after meal after snack after meal?

But the truth is, as you build awareness of your food habits and begin to see patterns in your eating, you will also begin to take more responsibility for your food choices.

It's worth repeating: hunger is caused by the interplay of internal and external triggers. We may not be completely aware of those triggers. We can't see them, whether they're the physiological actions of hormones and neurochemicals or emotional states like anxiety, stress, depression, boredom or loneliness. The external triggers may also act upon us in obscure or unconscious ways: the clock telling us it's dinnertime, the family sitting down at the big table, the sight or smell of food – even a photograph in a magazine or an advert on television.

By forcing you to pay attention to the feelings you have about food and eating, the food diary makes you aware of your own ability to make choices.

REMEMBER: NO DEPRIVATION AHEAD

A small percentage of people – knowing they are about to 'start a diet' – will eat everything under the sun. A kind of Last Supper mentality kicks in, as people binge on their favourite foods 'one last time'. Patients tell me they actually have Farewell to Food nights. Even before appearing in my office for the first time, they'll fill up on all the high-calorie foods they love. These foods, they're certain, I'll be asking them to abandon forever.

That Last Supper attitude is a tip-off to me that the individual is a chronic dieter who equates dieting with deprivation – and with failure. I try to impress on such a person that keeping a food diary is a tool, not a sign that deprivation is in his future.

The food diary is a tool of your own empowerment

More typically, my colleagues and I often find that the diaries of new patients don't quite match the information we gleaned in the intake interview. During the initial conversation, when we review a typical day's eating and try to understand the challenging times of day, people often overlook many of their snacks or impulsive buys.

It is human nature to try to look good, of course – and that could be one reason we don't get the whole story when we're asking people to work from memory. But I also think that even if you are trying to be honest, memory alone isn't enough. Before we can get a handle on our real relationships with food, we need to accurately record our eating habits. You need to have pen in hand and your diary ready for at least a few days.

THE DIARY: YOUR MIRROR

I know I need the accurate record of a diary to help people. And I believe you need it, too, if you're going to help yourself.

In addition to accuracy, responsibility for keeping the diary faithfully is essential. The attitude that the diary is 'just another chore – I'll catch up on it later' is a sure path to disaster. One of my patients, a busy executive, wanted to hand over the assignment to his wife and secretary. Since the secretary typically ordered his lunch and his wife invariably dined with him, he believed they would remember what he ate better than he did. Besides, he contended, he was a busy man, an important executive, somebody used to delegating tasks he didn't have time for. 'If you don't make the time to keep your food diary accurately and faithfully,' I told him, 'you're probably not ready to start a weight-loss programme.' He kept the diary religiously from that moment on.

For some people, the mere fact that they must answer to a piece of paper – the diary – is sufficient to raise their food awareness. The minute they know they have to write down what they're eating, forethought takes over – along with increased responsibility for the food choices they make.

This is the first step towards better choices

And choice, of course, is what this programme is about. It's about putting you in charge of your eating, changing your relationship with food without changing your lifestyle. The first step to that is mindfulness. That's what the food diary does and why its value is inestimable.

Now it's your turn.

HOW TO START

Draw out a chart with the same headings used in the diaries on the previous pages. Keep a copy with you at all times each day. For at least a week, record every bite and sip you take – with the exception of water and low-calorie beverages.

For the sake of accuracy, make sure you write down what you've had the minute you've eaten it. If you put off making the notation, you will almost certainly omit an important item in your diary entry.

Here's how to fill in each entry on the diary template:

■ **Time.** Record the exact time of day that you are eating.

■ **Food.** Note what you have eaten and how it was prepared, if applicable – in the case of chicken, for example, whether it was grilled, fried, steamed or roasted; and the size of the serving as best you can determine it. Describe as many ingredients in the dish as you think necessary – not just a roast chicken but a roast chicken stuffed with leeks and wild rice, or, in another example, not just a tuna sandwich but a tuna sandwich on wholemeal bread with lettuce, tomato and mayonnaise.

■ **Hunger Level.** For the purpose of this diary, I want you to define hunger as a desire to eat regardless of the reason. Rate the desire on a scale from 0 to 4, with zero indicating no hunger and 4 indicating extreme hunger.

■ **Situation (Place/Activity).** Where were you when you had the food or drink – bedroom, restaurant, kitchen, taxi, office – and in what situation – with a companion, reading a book, holding a meeting? This information is helpful because I don't want you to change your lifestyle, just your relationship with food.

■ **Comments.** Note anything you feel is relevant to your food choice or to the way you felt after eating. Some typical comments? 'That piece of cake was worth it for the calories'. . . 'It was foolish to eat those biscuits'. . . 'I was eating in someone's house and had no choice'.

EVALUATING YOUR FOOD DIARY

Did you recognise yourself in any of the classic eating profiles in this chapter? Chances are there were characteristics in all four that resonated with you, parts of each that struck you with a shock of recognition – whether you identified with the exact lifestyle or not. Now it's time to analyse your food diary to assess exactly what kind of relationship you have with food.

Some choices may be more 'typical' than you realised

After you have scrupulously kept your food diary for a week, sit down, look it over, and get ready to evaluate it. The notes you saw above – on Susan, Stan, Diana and Doug – are just the kinds of notes you want to make about yourself and your own eating habits. You're looking for patterns – recurring situations in which you make food choices. The diary helps you see where you've chosen a high-calorie option or the less-healthy alternative.

Some situations may sound just like something you've seen in the four classic eating profiles. Some choices may leap out at you as unnecessary – even inappropriate. That's precisely what you're looking for.

Let's take a look, item by item.

■ **Time.** Does the diary show that at certain times of the day you tend to eat more? Are other food choices available to you at those times?

If your diary shows that you have a late-afternoon craving for food pretty much every day, there are probably some foods you can keep on hand at home, in the office, even in your handbag or briefcase. Eating those foods might make more sense than getting items from the vending machine or the tea trolley or the ice-cream van.

■ **Food.** What kinds of choices do you usually make? Are you choosing mostly protein? Mostly starch? Or was it starch in the morning and protein in the afternoon?

Your food diary will show whether you eat lots of sweet foods or whether salt appeals to your taste. Once you know that, you can begin to think of lower-calorie options in the sweet or salty category.

■ **Degree of Hunger.** Does the diary show that you ate when you didn't feel truly hungry? Sometimes? Often?

Many people eat in response to feelings of boredom or tension. Did you eat for those reasons? If so, were you in touch with that feeling when you made your food choice?

■ **Situation (Place/Activity).** Can you find any connection between the situation in which you found yourself and the fact that you reached for food? Think about these entries a moment, and you may be able to see the connection between the situation and the kind of food you chose.

■ **Comments.** Explore what you wrote. What do your comments tell you about your eating habits? What do they reveal about your hunger?

Be honest and candid as you evaluate your food diary. Remember: this is an exercise in awareness. Nobody is asking you – now or ever – to change your eating habits or patterns in terms of when, why, or how you eat. The aim will be to find healthier, lower-calorie ways of working with those patterns. To get there, you must start with awareness.

WHY WRITING IT DOWN WORKS

'No need to write it down,' you say to yourself. 'I can keep my food diary in my head.'

Yes, but keeping a diary in your head isn't nearly as effective as putting things down on paper, as researchers in health psychology have conclusively demonstrated. According to a study at the Centre for Behavioural Medicine in Chicago, writing things down serves as 'a focusing device'. The requirements of keeping a food diary lends authority to the process itself and thus helps you pay closer attention to your eating.

Writing things down also increases your commitment by helping to turn an abstract, long-term goal into short-term reminders. The food diary 'helps create an internal dialogue', researchers say, in which you emphasise the importance of what you're doing.

Finally, writing down what you're eating lends an objective power to what you're doing: this is a problem you're solving, not a condition that makes you helpless.

The moral? Write it down – consistently, carefully, in black and white.

GETTING THE PICTURE

One picture is worth a thousand words, the ancient saying assures us. One of the most useful discoveries I've made during the years of my practice – and one of the most important aspects of the weight-loss programme I administer – is the importance of visual demonstration. A patient being treated for weight loss typically has weekly appointments, and each week, our nutrition-ist will prepare another demonstration for the patient. For example, perhaps we'll place a scone next to a plate of raisin bread and low-sugar jam that has the same number of calories (*see opposite*). Or a small portion of lemon tart next to seven scoops of lemon sorbet with an equivalent calorie count.

Whatever the specifics of the different demonstrations, one truth remains constant: the visual impact makes a difference. You can hear a message a million times, but when you see it demonstrated, it's really brought home.

SEEING FOR YOURSELF

That's why we're replicating the food demonstrations in the pages of this book, so you can see for yourself how wide-ranging your food options are, how easy it is to substitute one food for another and how great a difference it can make.

The pictures that follow are not trick photography. No closely guarded secrets lurk here. However, somewhere along the line, you'll be surprised. You'll see that a food you avoided because you thought it was 'fattening' is really a good choice for weight loss. Or that a food you believed was a good 'diet' choice is high in calories. For example, can it be true that a bowl of boiled sweets has no more calories than a small serving of nuts and dried fruit (*see page 73*)? Seeing is believing.

As you will realise by now, these pictures are designed to do more than work up your appetite. They show you exactly what your choices are and what the result will be when you decide to eat one food instead of another. Each of the portions shown is carefully measured. In each photograph, the food you're seeing has exactly the number of calories indicated. So you don't have to guess what someone means by 50 grams. Just remember these photographs in the course of a normal day, and you can make your choices the way people really do – without measuring spoons or scales or calorie-counter books.

In this chapter you'll see a lot of what seem like optical illusions. In some sections you'll see a large meal with relatively few calories. Other sections show the foods that would seem to be low-calorie but hide more calories than you can imagine. Throughout, we'll show you some of the many choices you can make when faced with decisions about what to eat.

HOW THE FOOD DEMONSTRATIONS WORK

Here's the way the food demonstrations are organised in the pages ahead:

■ **EQUAL CALORIES, DIFFERENT PORTIONS:** You'll learn how much more you can eat – and discover healthier choices – when you see the food images on these pages.

■ **EQUAL PORTIONS, DIFFERENT CALORIES:** Become an expert in making choices between the same quantities of the same types of foods. These images will help you become adept at selecting foods that may have one-half or one-third of the calories of the other selections.

■ **MORE FOOD FOR LESS CALORIES:** If you have a healthy appetite – and who doesn't? – you'll find that the foods in this section are worth learning off by heart. Why? Because you can eat more of these foods and get fewer calories than you'd get from smaller amounts of higher-calorie choices.

There's no right way to read these pictures. Whether they startle you or reinforce what you already knew, let them be your guide to making informed choices. True, all you have to do is look at these demonstrations, and you're likely to have a lasting memory of what they show you about food. On the other hand, it won't hurt to return to this chapter a few days or a few weeks from now, just to make sure you remember what you've seen – and to reinforce the low-calorie choices you'll be making now and in the future. And if these pictures start to make you hungry, they will also give you some good ideas about low-calorie ways to satisfy your hunger. It's all part of the process of Food Awareness Training.

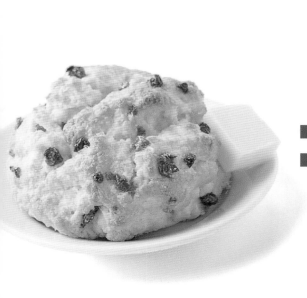

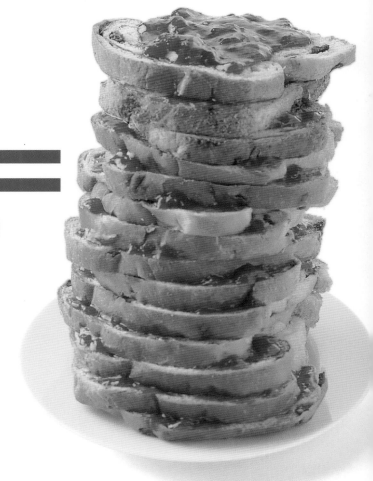

A scone with butter, or a whole stack of raisin bread with low-sugar jam? Believe it or not, both contain the same number of calories, and one is far more than you could eat at a sitting.

EQUAL CALORIES, DIFFERENT PORTIONS

BREAKFAST

This food demonstration tells the story in the form of a simple equation. The croissant looks innocent enough, but even without butter, it contains 250 calories.

Now look at the bigger picture to the right. All the fresh fruit you see plus the bread roll and jam adds up to the same number of calories as that croissant. And if you choose the fruit, you're getting more than just a good deal on calories. Fruit is a rich source of antioxidant vitamins and minerals.

'Choose the healthy option and you will be getting your recommended five daily servings of fruit and vegetables.'

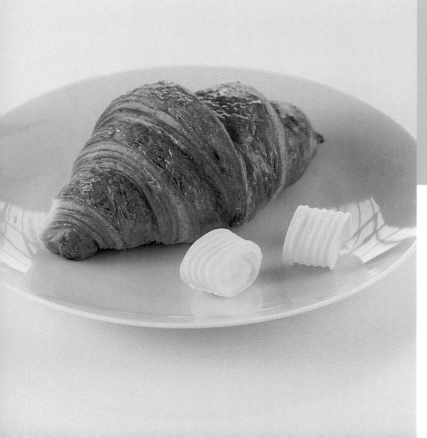

1 croissant (67g)
250 calories

+

2 butter curls (32g)
120 calories

---

370 calories

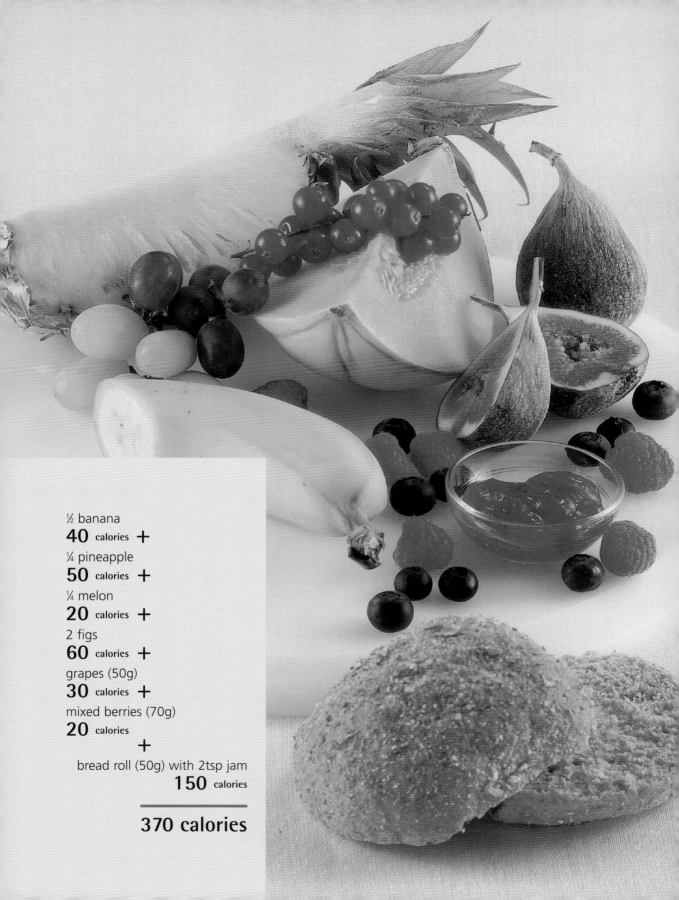

½ banana
40 calories **+**

¼ pineapple
50 calories **+**

¼ melon
20 calories **+**

2 figs
60 calories **+**

grapes (50g)
30 calories **+**

mixed berries (70g)
20 calories
+

bread roll (50g) with 2tsp jam
150 calories

370 calories

MID-MORNING SNACK

Our staff nutritionist says she has seen more people gain weight on low-fat snacks than on any other food. Take a look at the images below – can a banana and eight dried apricot halves really have the same calorie count as a reduced-fat snack bar? Yes. And the fruit contains fibre, vitamins and minerals, so it's a healthy option, too.

'Don't just go for the low-fat snack.'

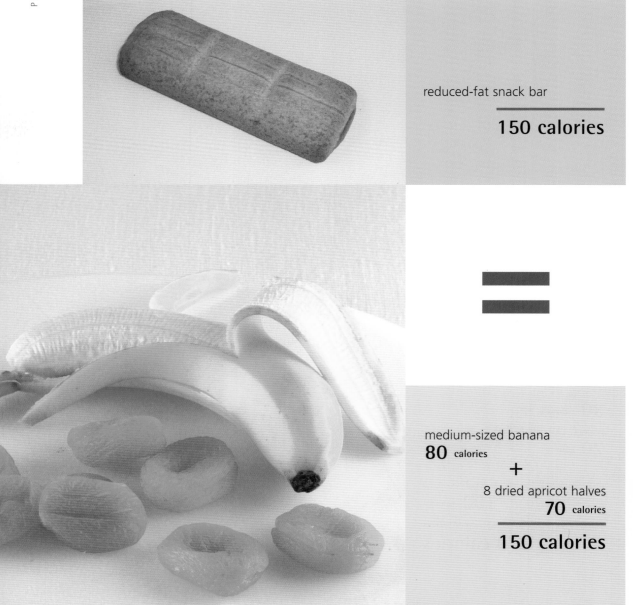

reduced-fat snack bar

150 calories

=

medium-sized banana
80 calories

+

8 dried apricot halves
70 calories

150 calories

Nuts and dried fruits are nutritious, healthy foods. But have a look at the comparison below. That single bowl of nuts and dried fruit contains 600 calories – the equivalent of a large bowl of boiled sweets!

One look at the sweets, and you may think you'll need to resist them with all the willpower at your command. These are forbidden foods, aren't they? Take a closer look. Surprisingly, the sweets are the calorie bargain. And sweets will last a long time, if you keep each one in your mouth, enjoying their flavour for a long time.

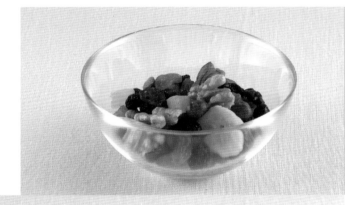

bowl of mixed nuts and dried fruit (100g)

600 calories

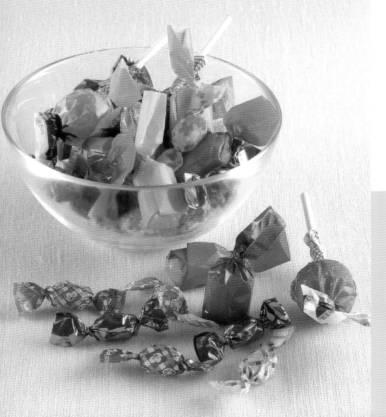

mix of boiled sweets (180g)

600 calories

STARTERS

Want to start your meal with a touch of class? Well, before you make your high-class choices, consider what you're seeing here. A piece of liver pâté on half a slice of toast contains 130 calories. But for the same calorie count, you could have a generous portion of smoked salmon, with succulent capers and cool cucumber instead.

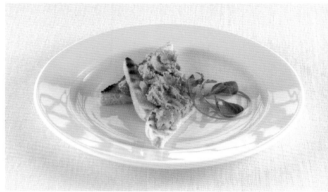

liver pâté (20g)
90 calories

+

half a slice of toast
40 calories

―――――――――――

130 calories

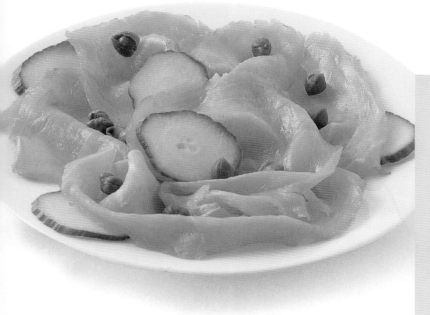

smoked salmon (90g) with capers and cucumber

―――――――――――

130 calories

Or maybe you'll opt for a small platter of charcuterie. But how about choosing something a little more luxurious and varied, with a whole range of tastes – salty, smooth, pungent and oily? Try smoked halibut and blinis topped with caviar and sour cream – you'll get a stylish, larger starter for the equivalent calorie count.

'Choose varied tastes and textures – enjoy your meal to the full!'

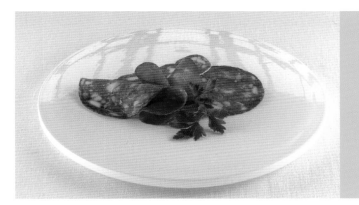

charcuterie platter (60g)

175 calories

=

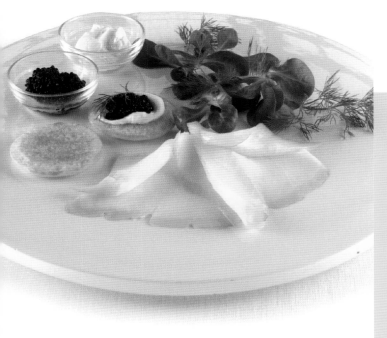

smoked halibut (30g)
40 calories **+**

2 blinis
60 calories **+**

caviar (20g)
60 calories **+**

sour cream (½ tbsp)
15 calories

175 calories

BITE-SIZED SNACK

Love cheese? Who doesn't? But the calorie content can make it a costly food. Here's a little image to keep in your memory bank. A single square of cheddar is not enough to satisfy a cheese craving, but it is the caloric equivalent of a bowl of soup. In addition, the bowl of soup offers a treasury of nutrition.

'Cheese is a high calorie snack.'

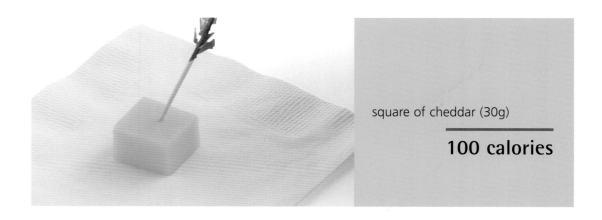

square of cheddar (30g)

100 calories

=

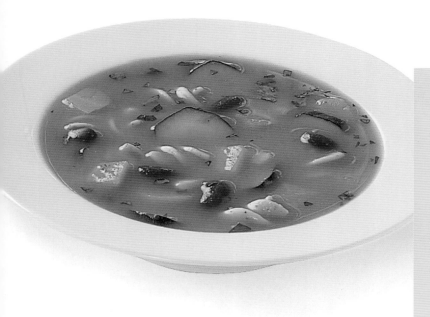

chunky vegetable soup (200ml)

100 calories

Want a bite of bacon cheeseburger? Go ahead, but there's a cost. There are 220 calories in this bite. If you were to eat the whole burger, it would cost you 660 calories – not to mention all the saturated fats and cholesterol you'd be taking in.

The alternative is just as easy. Why not choose a soya-based veggie burger instead? For the equivalent calorie count as a third of a bacon cheeseburger, you can enjoy the whole veggie burger, guilt-free. In fact, the veggie burger is thoroughly good for you.

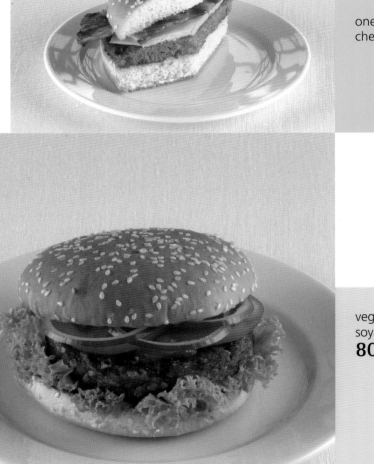

one-third of a quarter-pounder cheeseburger with bacon

220 calories

veggie burger:
soya burger (60g)
80 calories **+**
bun (50g)
120 calories **+**
lettuce, tomato, onion and relish
20 calories

220 calories

MEAT OR FISH?

When you are dining out, it can be hard to resist traditional fare on the menu, such as steak and chips. You know it will be tasty and nutritious, and that you will leave the table feeling full and satisfied.

But take a moment to compare that dish with the feast opposite – a slap-up meal, including a side salad, a dessert and a glass of wine for the same calorie count. Perhaps you'll change your order?

'A plate of steak and chips has the equivalent calorie count of a three-course meal.'

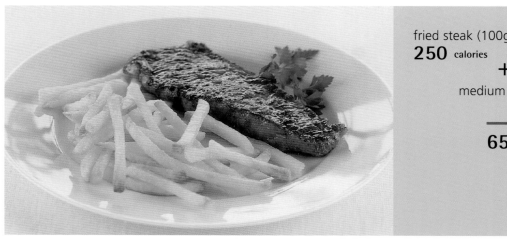

fried steak (100g)
250 calories

+

medium portion of fries
400 calories
_____

650 calories

'A luxurious meal doesn't have
to be a high-calorie option.'

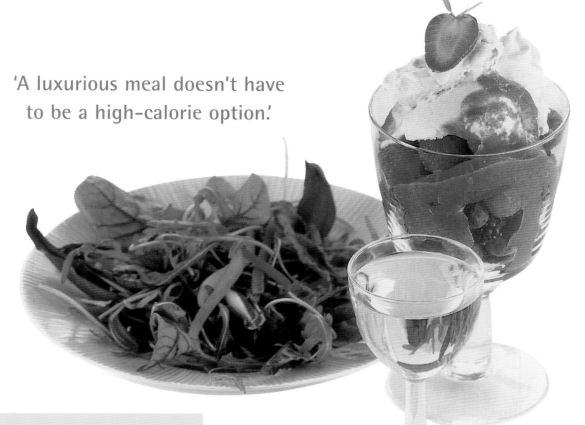

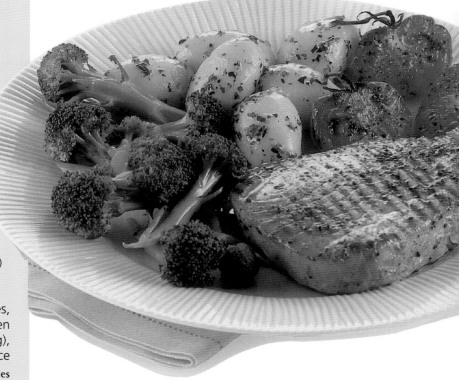

chargrilled tuna (200g) with
lemon garnish
200 calories **+**

herby new potatoes (150g)
110 calories **+**

broccoli (50g)
20 calories **+**

grilled tomatoes (100g)
20 calories **+**

salad with red and yellow
pepper garnish
30 calories **+**

a glass of white wine (150ml)
100 calories **+**

mixed berries,
topped with strawberry frozen
yoghurt (100g),
cream and drizzle sauce
170 calories

_____

650 calories

BARBECUE

It's a friend's birthday party and you're having an evening barbecue. But how can you enjoy the feast, let your hair down and still keep the calorie count low? Before you choose the seemingly obvious low-fat option, have a look at the pictures shown here. Instead of the two low-fat sausages and the two mouthfuls of garlic bread, you could have the platter of prawns, mushrooms, baked potato, vegetables and all that watermelon. The calorie count is equivalent.

'You might think that choosing low-fat sausages will be the best choice for your waist-line – but seafood and vegetables will still offer fewer calories than the supposedly "low-fat" option.'

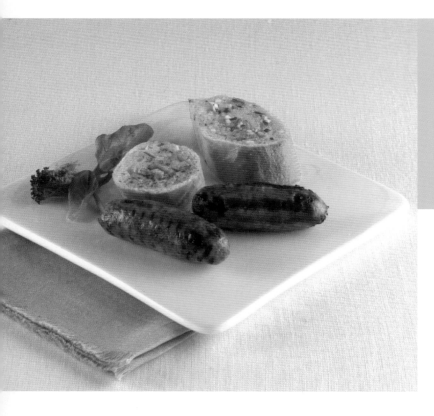

2 low-fat sausages (100g)
180 calories

+

garlic bread (50g)
200 calories

___

380 calories

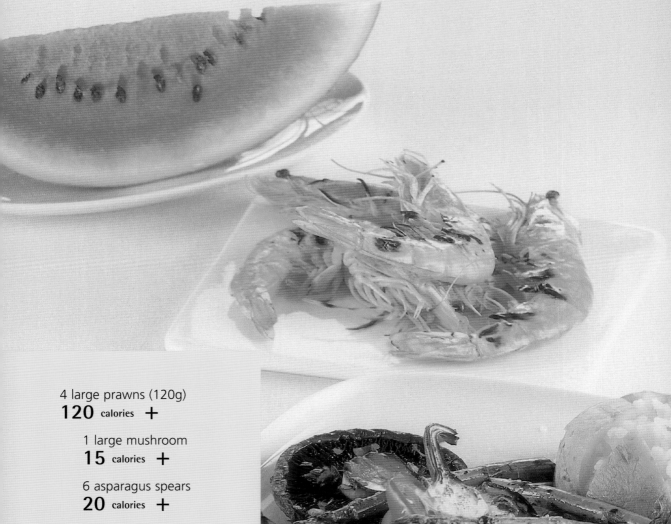

4 large prawns (120g)
120 calories **+**

1 large mushroom
15 calories **+**

6 asparagus spears
20 calories **+**

red pepper (80g)
30 calories **+**

onion (80g)
25 calories **+**

large baked potato
120 calories **+**

1 large slice of watermelon
50 calories

---

380 calories

SIDE ORDERS

We all know rice is good for us. It's the world's 'basic food', after all. Unfortunately, we underestimate the calories in steamed rice more than any other starch. The next time you reach for the rice, think again. One portion of rice has 320 calories, which is the same calorie count as that large dish of tasty, mixed vegetables shown below.

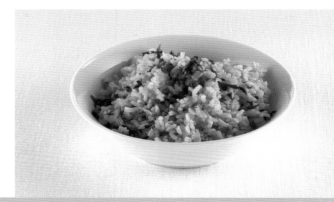

bowl of plain
brown rice (230g)

320 calories

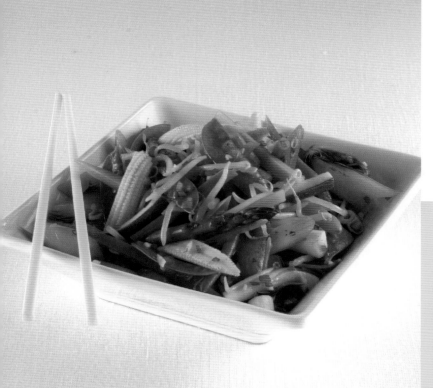

dish of mixed stir-fried
vegetables (600g)

320 calories

FRIED OR BAKED?

Any fried food is high in fat. In fact, there's so much fat in these fries that you'll probably consume more calories from the frying fat than from the potato. How about three baked potatoes and ratatouille instead? The calories are equivalent. And if you eat just two potatoes, you'll be cutting your calorie intake by a third.

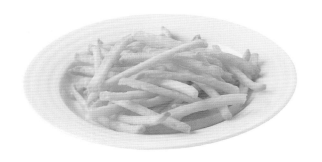

medium portion
of fries (110g)

400 calories

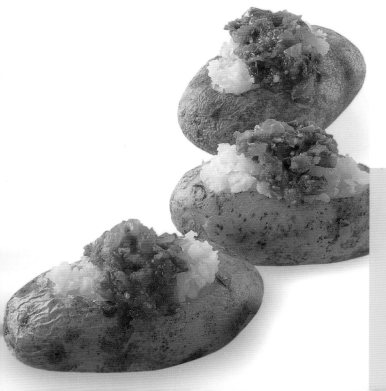

3 small baked potatoes
360 calories
+
ratatouille (60g)
40 calories

400 calories

VEAL OR POULTRY?

Veal may seem like a healthier, lower-calorie option in comparison to other red meats, such as beef or lamb. But once it's been dipped in batter and fried into a piece of wienerschnitzel, this choice on the menu can really increase your calorie intake, even if you only have a modest portion. And that's not even mentioning the saturated fat.

If you're in the mood for meat, you can eat almost twice the amount for the same number of calories. Just look at the marinated turkey and vegetable skewers shown opposite and then take your pick.

'Turkey and vegetable kebabs are a healthy meal. You can have a sizeable portion and still keep the calories down.'

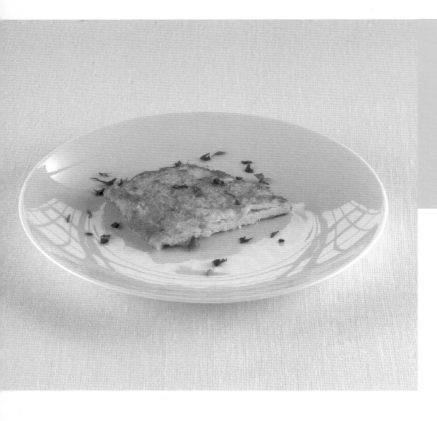

wienerschnitzel (65g)

190 calories

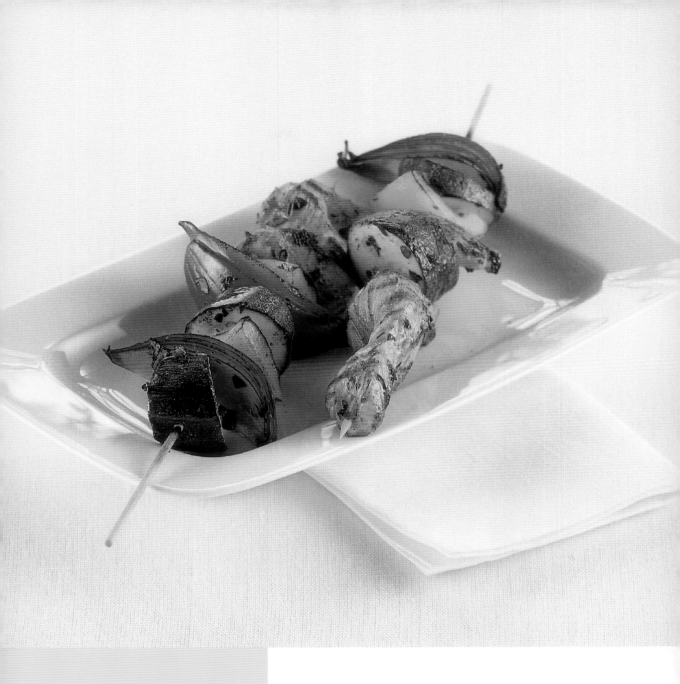

2 marinated turkey (125g) and
vegetable skewers

190 calories

'Grilled foods are better for your
weight than foods that have been
fried or baked in oil.'

STREET FOOD

When you're in a hurry, it's easy to grab a quick snack to eat on the run. But you should still consider the choices available to you. If you love hot dogs, the one frankfurter below probably won't be enough for you. But look at what you could have instead.

You could have three falafals in a pitta bread, with salad and tasty raita for the equivalent number of calories that you find in the hot dog. And since the protein in the falafal is from a vegetable rather than an animal source, it's the healthier option, too.

'If you're weight- and health-conscious, you might want to pass the hot-dog stand and head for the nearest take-away selling falafals instead.'

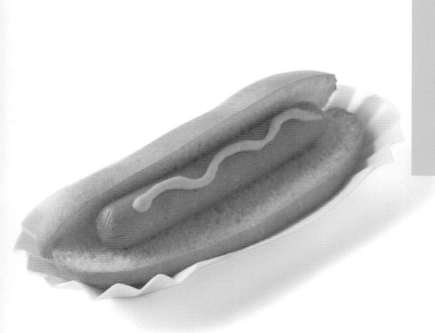

hotdog with mustard

360 calories

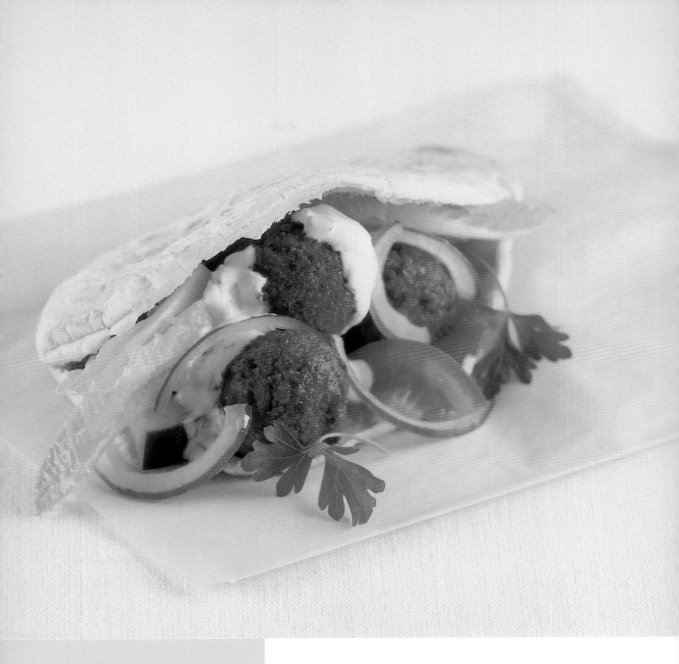

3 falafal balls (70g)
180 calories
+

pitta bread
150 calories
+

salad and raita
30 calories
_____

360 calories

WINTER WARMER

On cold winter evenings, it can be tempting to treat yourself to nourishing, creamy meals that make you feel warm and full. All those old favourites your mum used to cook you – like shepherd's pie or lasagne – are real comfort foods. Shame about the calories.

Even if you're watching your weight, though, you don't need to deprive yourself. Compare the two winter dishes shown here. For one small slice of lasagne, you could enjoy a large bowl of cassoulet and some french bread – all for the same calorie count.

'Comfort meals don't have to be calorie-ladden – bean and sausage cassoulet is brimming with nutrients, and will leave you feeling full.'

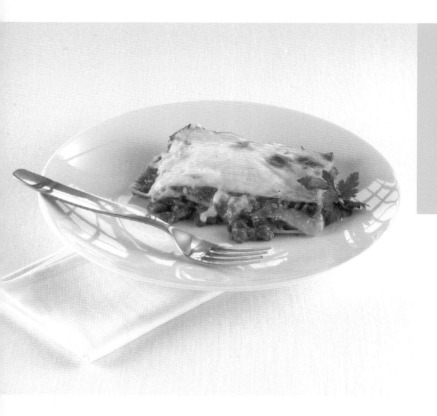

small lasagne (300g)

600 calories

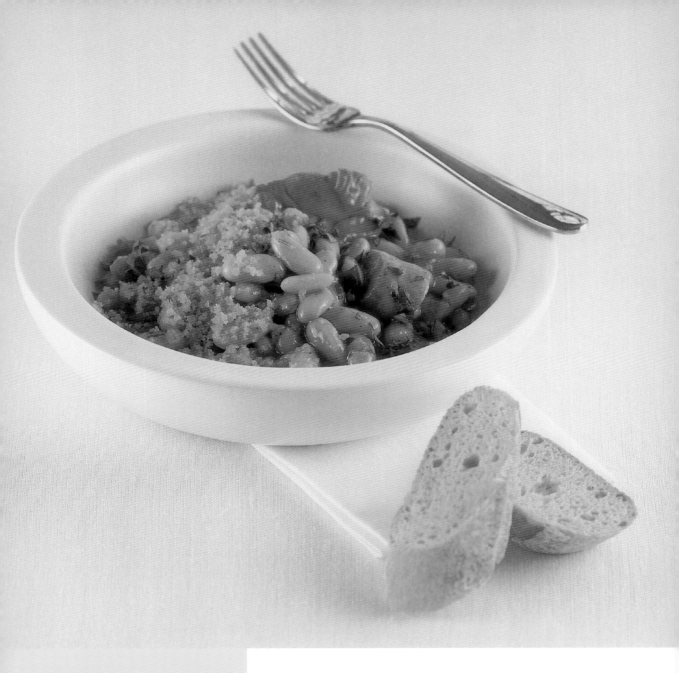

sausage and bean
cassoulet (400g)
500 calories

two 1-inch slices of french stick
100 calories
_____

600 calories

PASTRY

A fruit tart seems innocent enough compared to a dessert like cheesecake or chocolate-layer cake. However, if that's your view, it might be time for a tart reassessment. Take a look at the pictures here.

'You can eat 6 bowls of raspberries for the same calorie cost as one small raspberry tart.'

A fruit tart is made with a pastry that's so high in fat and sugar that it takes 6 bowls of fresh raspberries with whipped cream to equal a single raspberry tart. If you want the tart, by all means have it – but not because it's a low-calorie dessert. For a low-calorie raspberry taste, feast on raspberries – the real thing!

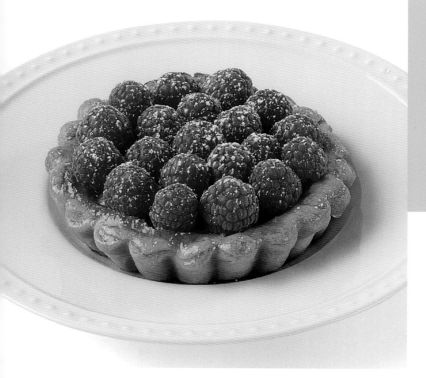

fruit tart (100g)

440 calories

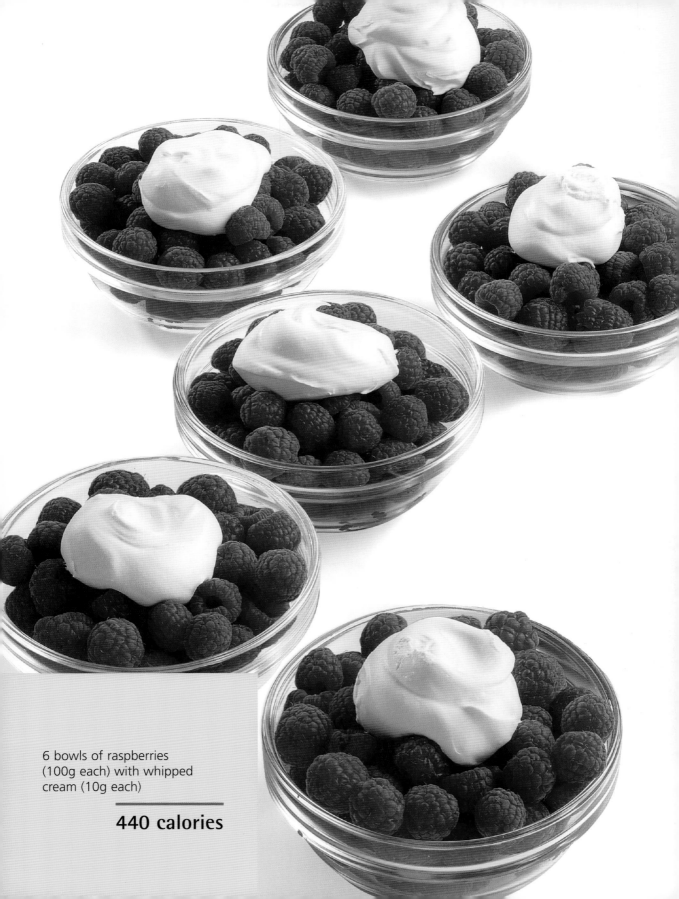

6 bowls of raspberries
(100g each) with whipped
cream (10g each)

440 calories

CHEESE OR DESSERT?

After a big meal, you might decide to forego your dessert and just have a modest little serving of cheese and a biscuit – just to round off the meal and keep the dessert-eaters company.

You see the cheese and crackers shown below? They contain as many calories as two waffles with berries and syrup topping. Which would you choose?

'Choosing that deliciously decadent dessert instead of foregoing it for a bite or two of cheese may – surprisingly – keep your calorie intake lower.'

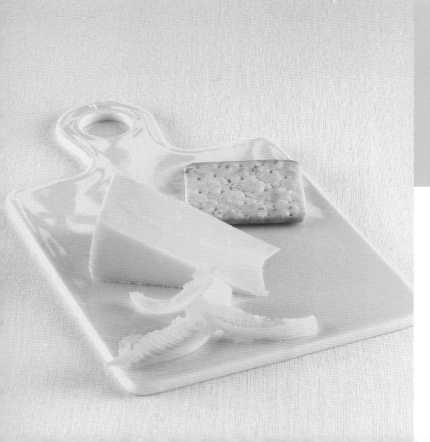

cheese (100g)
400 calories

+

1 cracker
50 calories

450 calories

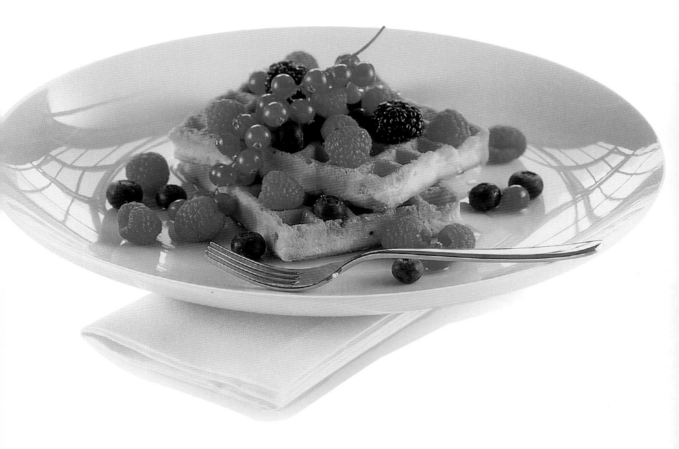

2 waffles
300 calories

+

syrup (3 tbsp)
100 calories

+

berries (175g)
50 calories

———————————

450 calories

DESSERT

If you think this one lonely crêpe and scoop of vanilla ice cream doesn't look like much for dessert, you're right. It isn't. And it will probably leave you wanting another helping. The choice on the right should give you something to consider.

'If you've got a sweet tooth, choose your dessert carefully, and then let go of your guilt complex.'

For the same number of calories, you could eat three sundaes, each containing sorbet, fresh fruit, whipped cream and sauce. Who doesn't love a sundae? But you'll probably be hard pressed to eat all three in one sitting, and just eating one will mean your calorie count will be even lower.

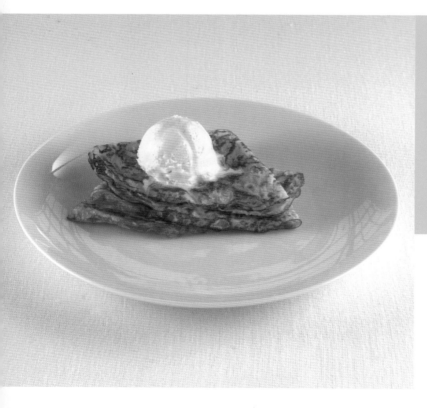

crêpe (100g)
280 calories **+**

scoop of vanilla
ice cream (60g)
100 calories **+**

syrup (2 tbsp)
70 calories

450 calories

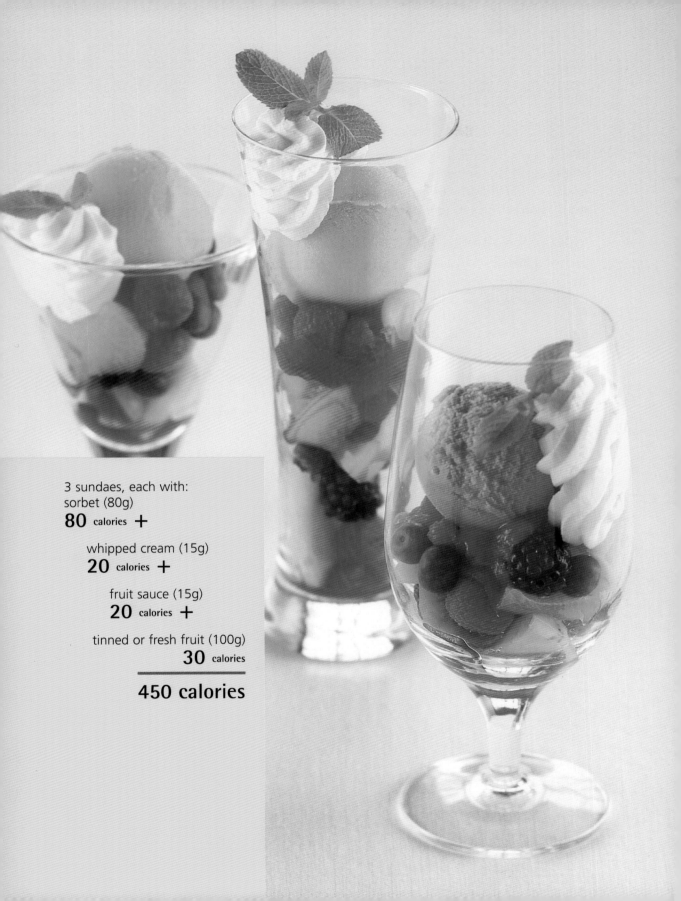

3 sundaes, each with:
sorbet (80g)
80 calories **+**

whipped cream (15g)
20 calories **+**

fruit sauce (15g)
20 calories **+**

tinned or fresh fruit (100g)
30 calories
_____

450 calories

TAPAS

When you're with friends for a night out at a tapas bar, it's easy to snack on all the dishes that are put in front of you. The choice of delicacies on offer can be huge, and because the portions seem small, it can be tempting to throw calorie-counting to the wind.

Take a closer look at what's on offer – you may be surprised by the calorie difference between dishes. For example, a portion of tortilla contains almost double the calories of eight garlic prawns, whereas the spicy mushrooms are a bargain for the weight-conscious.

'Don't forget to account for the calories you're taking in when you drink alcohol, too.'

spicy marinated
button mushrooms (50g)
with rosemary

25 calories

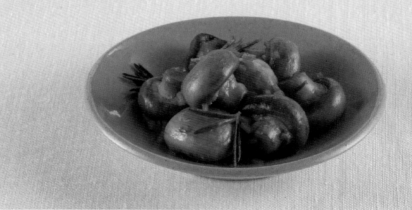

10 stuffed olives

60 calories

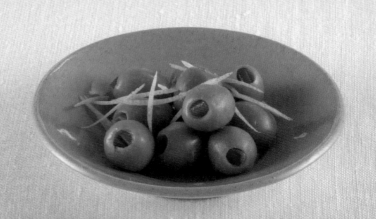

Sherry (50ml)

60 calories

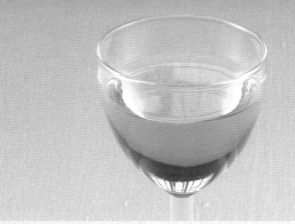

8 garlic prawns (60g)

100 calories

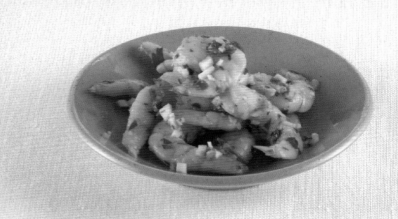

chorizo sausage (40g)

150 calories

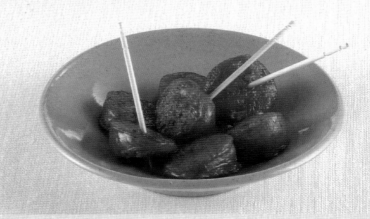

tortilla (90g)

180 calories

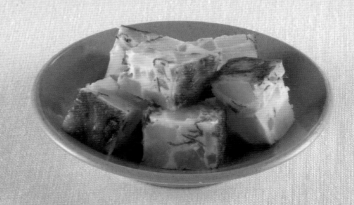

SALAD BAR

The variety on offer in a salad bar can leave you dithering between choices. But when you look at the difference in the calorie counts, you may find your choice becomes all too obvious.

It's easy to think of salads as the low-calorie option, but as you can see, that's not always the case. Next time you find yourself at your favourite salad bar, keep these pictures in mind.

'Try and avoid salads with rich, creamy dressings and vinaigrettes – that's where the calories are lurking.'

green salad and tomato

40 calories

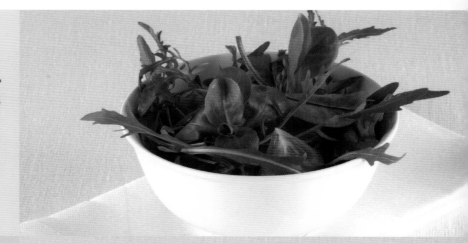

beetroot and orange salad

80 calories

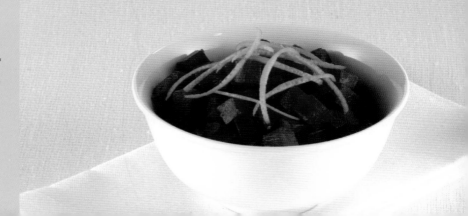

coleslaw
150 calories

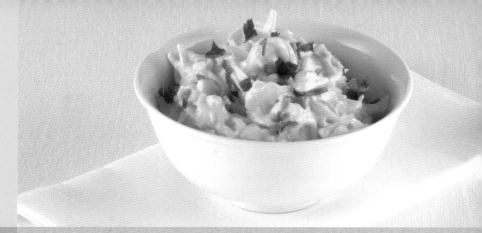

mixed bean salad
180 calories

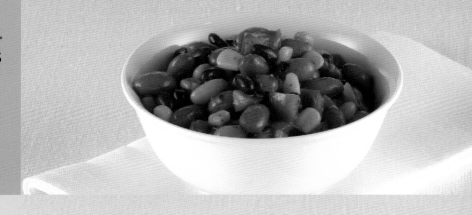

potato salad
300 calories

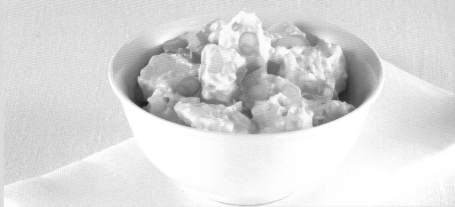

creamy pasta salad
400 calories

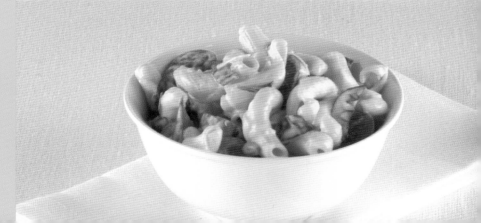

BREAD BASKET

Do you always take the bread roll offered at the restaurant? Do you eat bread daily? If so, you might want to spend some time contemplating the pictures below. As you can see, one bagel has as many calories as 5 slices of pumpernickel bread. It has more than twice as many calories as a small, wholemeal roll. Don't forget this visual advice on how to get the most bread for the fewest calories.

1 slice of pumpernickel

50 calories

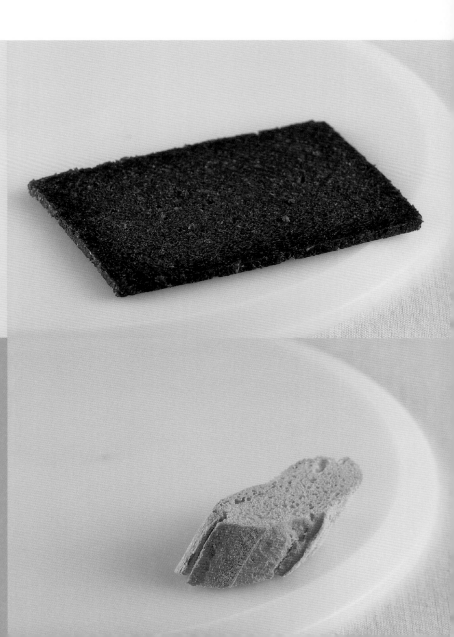

One 1-inch slice of french stick

50 calories

1 small wholemeal roll
(40g)
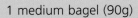
100 calories

1 pitta
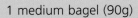
150 calories

1 medium bagel (90g)

250 calories

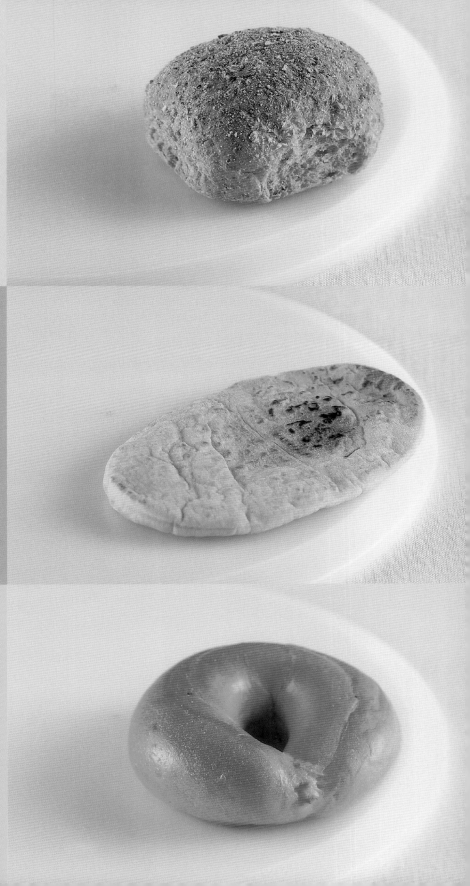

FAST FOOD

Sometimes, fast food is the only thing that will hit the spot and sometimes, despite all your good intentions, there's just no other option available. Then, since you're at the fast-food counter anyway, it's easy to let your weight-watching fall by the wayside as you blow out on all the high-calorie options on the menu. Instead of choosing that milkshake, which you're ordering just for the sake of it, why not opt for a thirst-quenching diet cola? Or choose a healthy beanburger instead of a quarter pounder with cheese – you'll still save calories.

'Even when you're eating fast food, the choices you make can affect your calorie intake dramatically.'

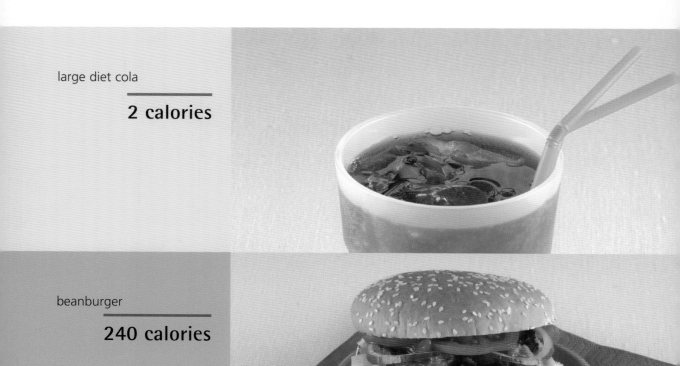

large diet cola

2 calories

beanburger

240 calories

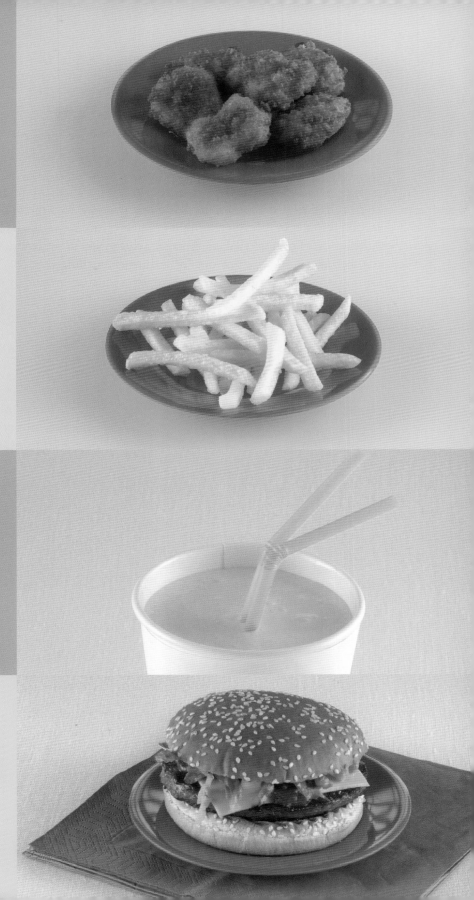

6 chicken nuggets

250 calories

medium fries (110g)

400 calories

medium milkshake

400 calories

quarter pounder with cheese

520 calories

INDIAN

Indian food offers a range of contrasts in tastes, textures and calories. Here are equal portions of lamb biryani and tandoori prawns, but each with vastly different fat and calorie contents. The lamb biriyani – cooked with raisins, coconut and ghee – is high in saturated fats and contains 800 calories. Tandoori prawns with vegetables and a savoury marinade, is low in fat and high in good protein from seafood, and it has less than half the calories of the lamb.

'Choose your side dish carefully, and you can cut your calorie intake in half.'

And as for the side dishes, spiced, Indian fried bread – keema paratha – has so many calories that it's the equivalent of a full meal. A single serving of keema paratha equals 330 calories, as opposed to a delicious tasting chickpea and spinach curry, at 120 calories.

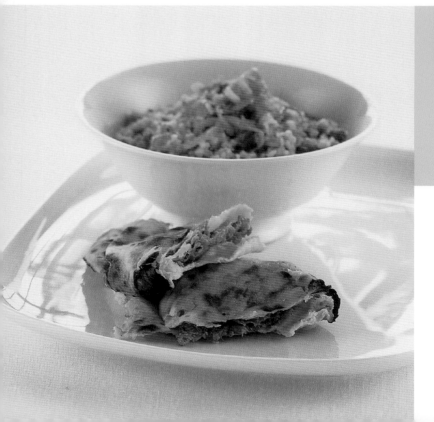

lamb biriyani (450g)
800 calories

+

keema paratha (100g)
330 calories

1130 calories

VS

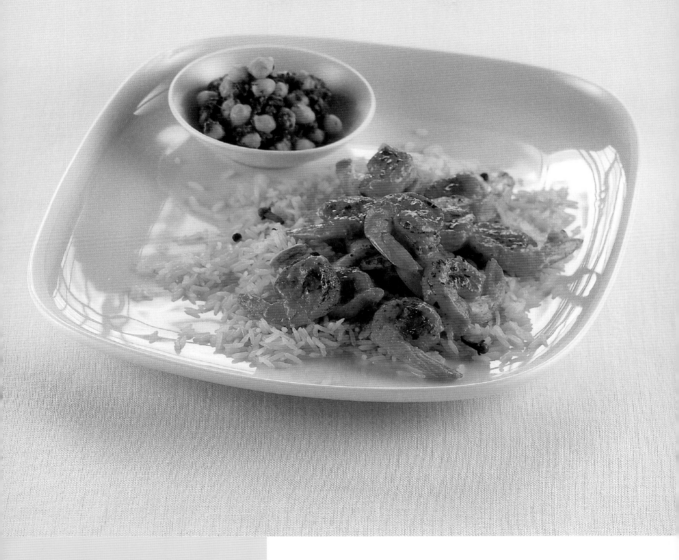

tandoori prawns (200g)
on a bed of boiled
pilau rice (120g)
400 calories
+
chickpea and spinach
curry (80g)
120 calories

520 calories

JAPANESE

Here are three classic Japanese dishes in equal portions – chicken tempura, shrimp teriyaki and sushi/sashimi. However, when you see equal portions, you can't automatically assume equal calories. Although the portions of teriyaki and sushi/sashimi have relatively low calorie counts, the tempura has double the amount.

'Cut down on deep-fried foods.'

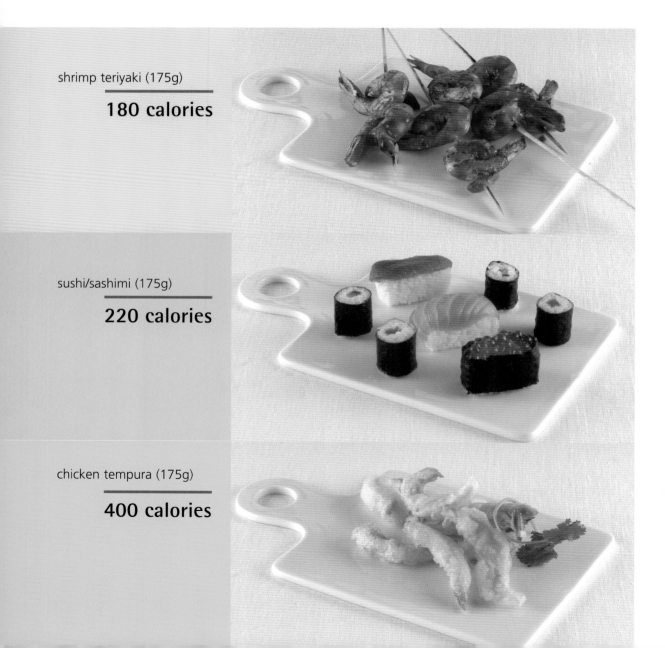

shrimp teriyaki (175g)

180 calories

sushi/sashimi (175g)

220 calories

chicken tempura (175g)

400 calories

MEXICAN

These two offerings both look enticing, but they boast substantially different calorie counts. One is a burrito stuffed with meat, cheese and sour cream – containing 760 calories. But now look at the alternative. Salsa prawns with lots of beans, rice and salad – containing about half the calories of the first option.

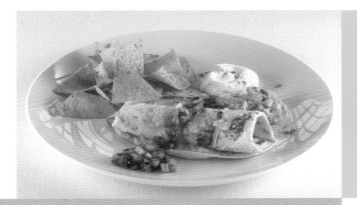

10-inch burrito with mince, cheese, sour cream, beans, salsa, guacamole (75g), tortilla chips (50g)

760 calories

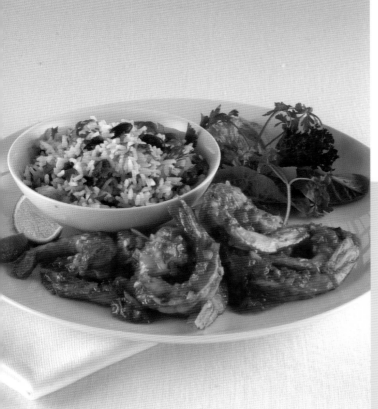

VS

salsa prawns (200g)
150 calories
+
beans (50g) and rice (150g)
200 calories
+
salad garnish
5 calories

355 calories

THAI

Thai food is delicious and distinctive, but if you are conscious of your weight, you need to make the right choices. Compare the calorie counts of three Thai fish cakes with three chicken satays.

'Thai food offers a wide array of lower-calorie choices, but be careful what you choose.'

steamed mushrooms
(100g)

100 calories

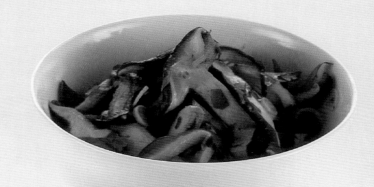

sour prawn soup (200ml)

130 calories

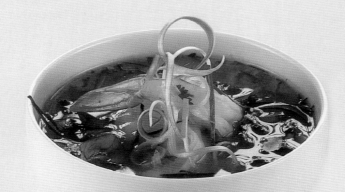

3 fish cakes with
sweet chilli sauce

150 calories

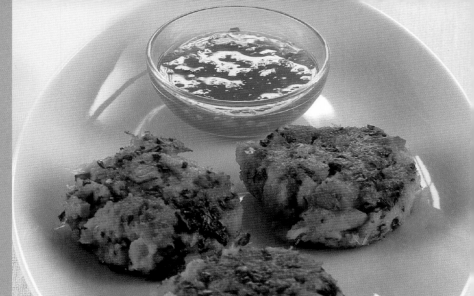

green chicken curry (200g)

300 calories

chicken satay (200g)

300 calories

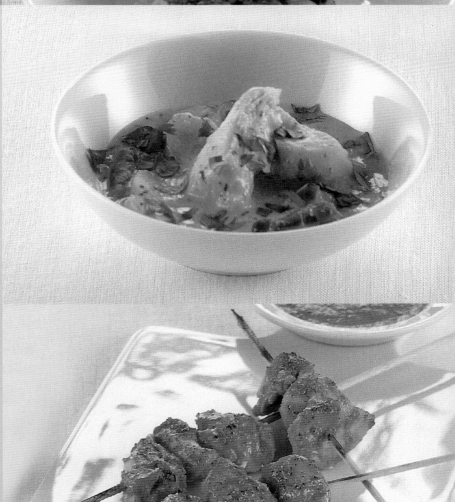

PIZZA

No, pizza isn't roulette. But there are low-calorie bets as well as high-calorie ones on the pizza wheel pictured here. Traditional mozzarella and tomato pizza, not to mention cheese and pepperoni, hold no surprises: they're high in calories.

Vegetable pizza, on the other hand, is a calorie bargain, as is a slice with tomato sauce and seafood (no cheese). Add the nutritional power of these two pizza slices, and the bargain gets even better.

'Order your pizza without cheese topping, or choose one that has plenty of vegetables on it, rather than meat.'

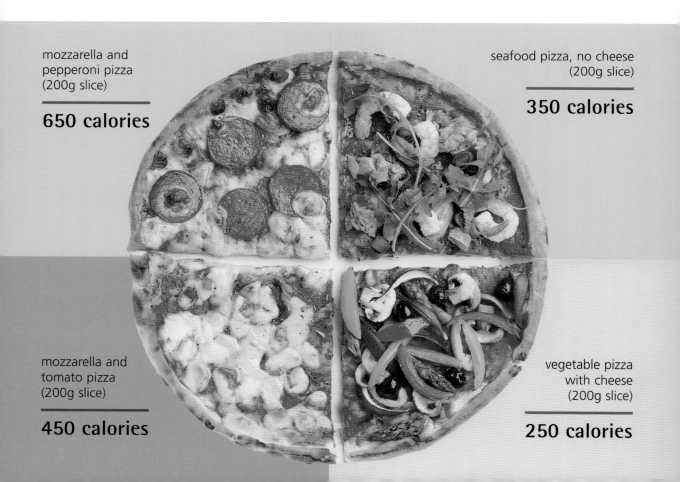

mozzarella and
pepperoni pizza
(200g slice)

650 calories

seafood pizza, no cheese
(200g slice)

350 calories

mozzarella and
tomato pizza
(200g slice)

450 calories

vegetable pizza
with cheese
(200g slice)

250 calories

POTATOES

Potatoes are a nutritious, healthy food. However, how they have been prepared can make a big difference to their fat content. Different types of potato dish can have widely differing calorie counts. Look at the comparison below.

'If you're trying to lose weight, avoid eating potatoes roasted or sautéed in oil.'

For instance, boiled potatoes have at least half the calorie count of roasted or sautéed potatoes. Even mashed potatoes, made with butter and milk, offer a significantly lower calorie count than these two high-calorie options.

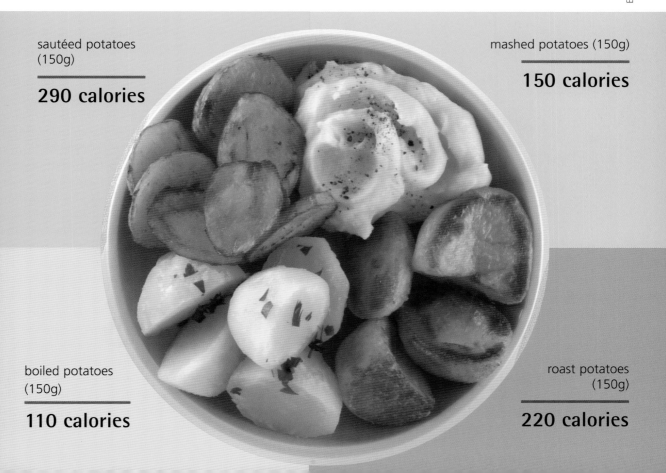

sautéed potatoes
(150g)

290 calories

mashed potatoes (150g)

150 calories

boiled potatoes
(150g)

110 calories

roast potatoes
(150g)

220 calories

MORE FOOD FOR LESS CALORIES

GREEK

Greek cuisine offers a range of exciting tastes. You can experience a slice of one of them – moussaka – for 560 calories. But is that really what you feel like?

Before you decide, picture the delights you could eat instead – and for fewer calories. The whole meal's worth of Greek food, shown right, offers plenty of tastes and textures – dolmades, baked prawns, tzatziki and melitzanosalata, topped off with some figs and a glass of retsina – all for a total of 490 calories.

'Enjoy all the delicious flavours of a whole Greek feast, instead of one slice of moussaka.'

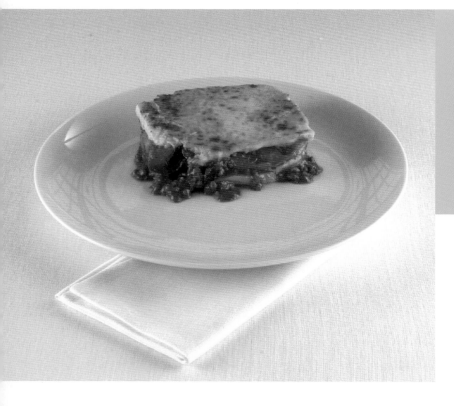

slice of moussaka (350g)

560 calories

VS

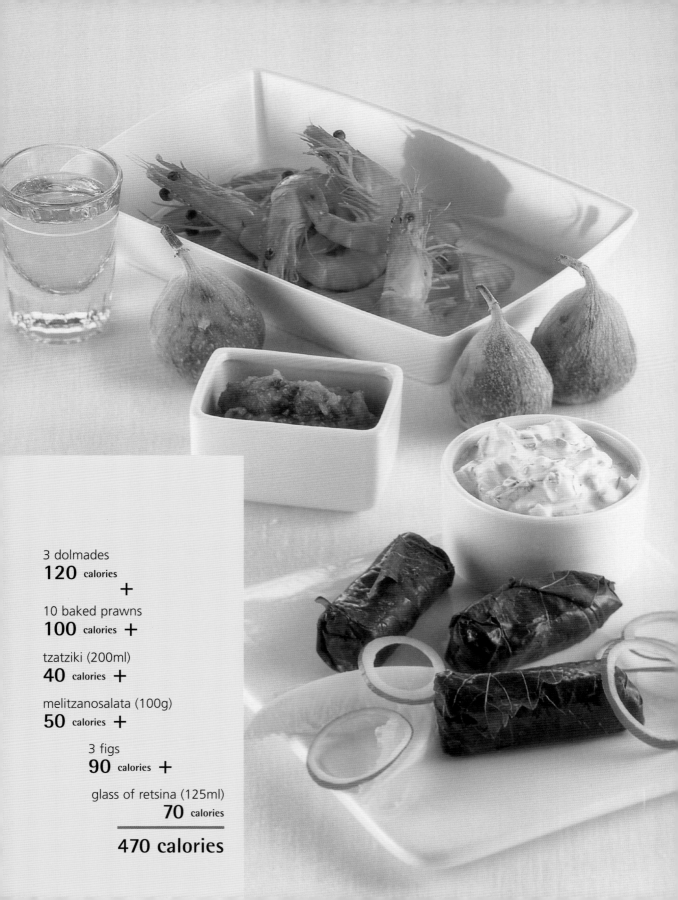

3 dolmades
120 calories
+

10 baked prawns
100 calories **+**

tzatziki (200ml)
40 calories **+**

melitzanosalata (100g)
50 calories **+**

3 figs
90 calories **+**

glass of retsina (125ml)
70 calories

470 calories

CHINESE

If you ate the whole meal pictured opposite, you would leave the table feeling satisfied. Amazingly, it has fewer calories than one of the starters below – the spring rolls or the small portion of spare ribs.

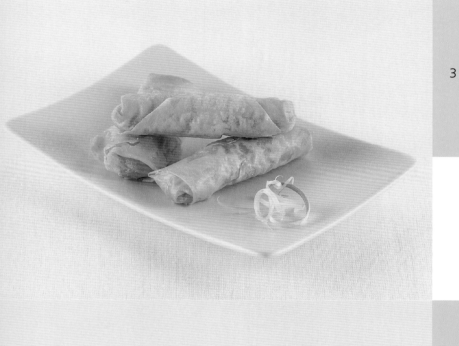

3 spring rolls (60g each)

500 calories

or

spare ribs (200g)

500 calories

VS

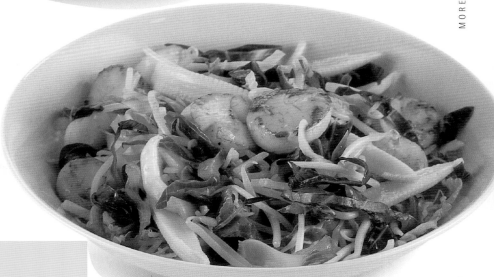

'Will you
choose one
starter, or a
whole meal?'

stir-fried scallops and Chinese
vegetables (350g)
320 calories
+
boiled rice (70g)
100 calories
+
Chinese vegetable soup
40 calories
_____
460 calories

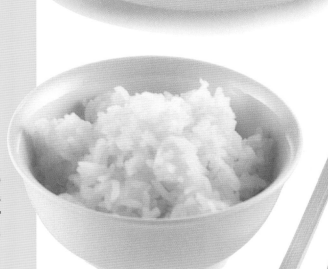

PASTA

Who could feel deprived eating the plate of pasta below, with its delicious creamy mushroom and bacon topping?

But before you say, 'I want more', take a look at the mouth-watering food that's shown in the meal opposite – and then consider your choices. The tomato and olive pasta dish is accompanied by a crunchy green salad, and followed by a fresh fruit salad and a scoop of sorbet. And all for fewer calories than the dish of creamy pasta. Which would you choose?

'You don't have to forego a side dish or a dessert if you choose your main dish carefully.'

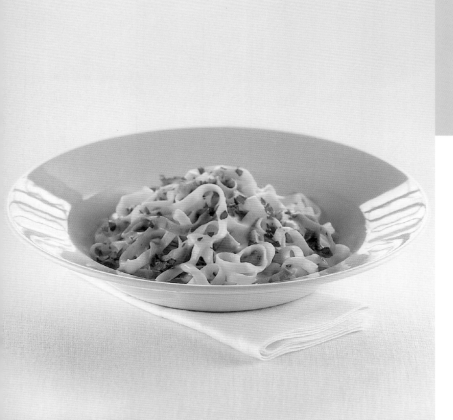

tagliatelle with cream, mushrooms and bacon (400g)

600 calories

VS

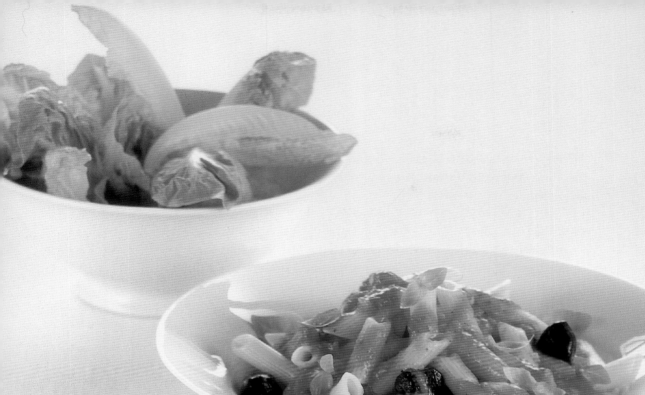
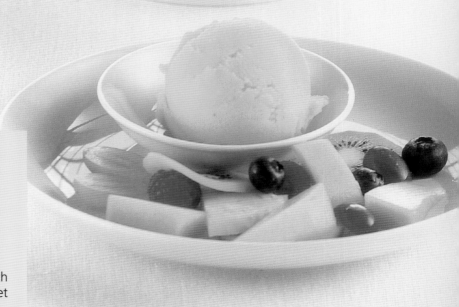

pasta with tomatoes and
olives (400g)
400 calories **+**

green salad
20 calories **+**

fresh fruit salad (50g) with
one scoop of sorbet
100 calories

_____

520 calories

PIZZA PLUS

A couple of slices of pizza? Well, maybe that's all you need. But next time you order the second slice, you may want to conjure up the image shown on the left.

Instead of two slices of pizza, you might prefer just one slice along with a generous serving of salad and a relaxing glass of white wine. In short, you'll get fewer calories from this meal with nearly a full day's supply of vitamins, minerals and fibre thrown in, too.

'More food for less is always a good bargain, especially when you can also get more food with more nourishment and fewer calories.'

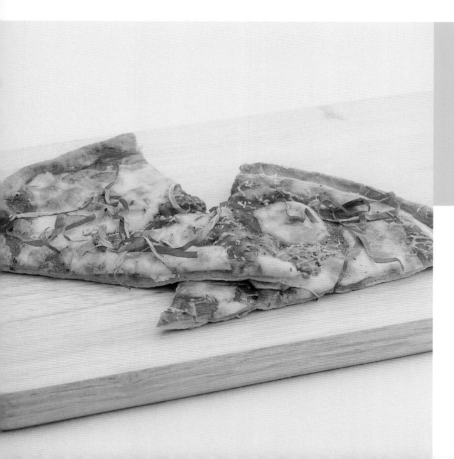

2 slices of cheese and tomato pizza (200g each)

900 calories

VS

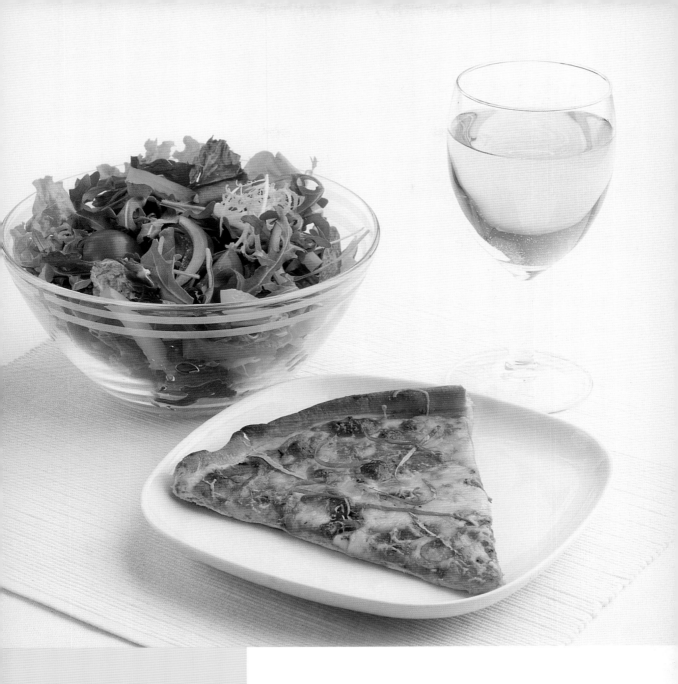

1 slice of cheese and
tomato pizza (200g)
450 calories **+**

salad
30 calories **+**

glass of white wine (125ml)
100 calories
───────────────
580 calories

'The equivalent of a light
snack can be transformed into a
satisfying meal.'

SALAD

You might have a weakness for cheese, but compare these two salads. You could have the small serving of goat's cheese salad, but you will still be hungry when you've finished it. Why not opt for the large crab salad instead? This option is not only filling, but think of all those beneficial seafood–nutrients, too.

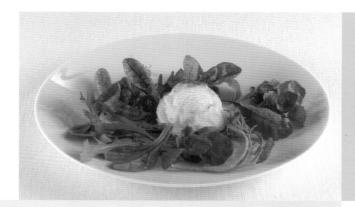

small toasted goat's cheese
salad (100g)

300 calories

VS

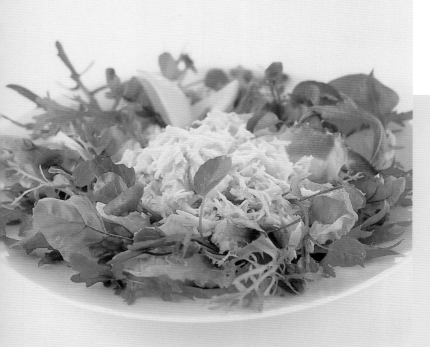

large crab salad

200 calories

DINNER

A cheese omelette is quick and easy to prepare, but for just a little more effort, you could enjoy a hearty meal such as chicken casserole, with plenty of healthy vegetables. Not only would this provide you with lots of different flavours, textures and nutrients, it would add fewer calories to your count.

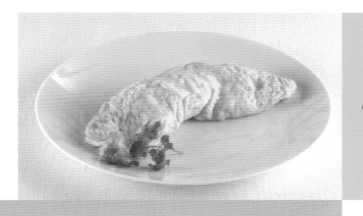

cheese omelette

490 calories

VS

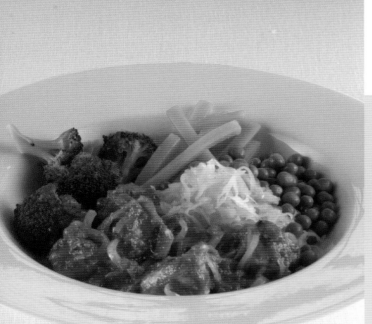

casseroled chicken breast (120g)
in tomato gravy
260 calories **+**
sauerkraut (50g)
10 calories **+**
peas (60g)
40 calories **+**
carrots (50g)
20 calories **+**
broccoli (50g)
20 calories

350 calories

STARTER OR MAIN COURSE?

Wolf down this small amount of prosciutto and melon or even the more filling portion of bruschetta – bread drizzled with olive oil and tomato – and you will barely take the edge off your appetite.

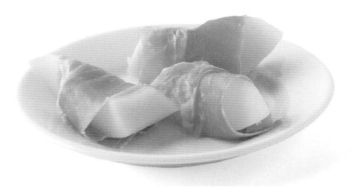

melon and prosciutto (120g)

330 calories

Yet if you eat either starter, you will have already taken in 330 calories before you have even tucked into your main course.

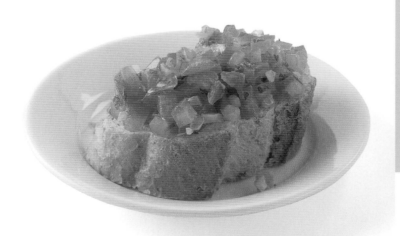

tomato bruschetta (90g)

330 calories

VS

But here's another picture to keep in mind. Contrast those small starters with this hefty bowl of moules marinière.

Look at the portion size! And yet the calorie count is only 250. Plus, you're getting a lot more nutrition with the mussels.

'Mussels are a great low-fat source of protein and minerals.'

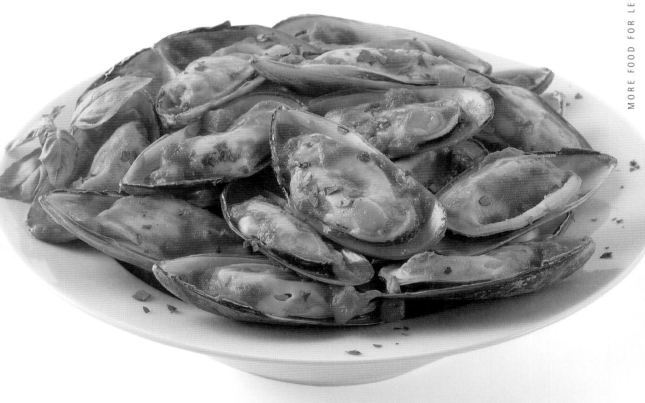

moules marinière (300g)

250 calories

PASTRY – YES OR NO?

When you are trying to lose weight, it's always difficult to decide whether to have a starter, or whether to forego the starter and save yourself for the dessert instead. That way, you're still watching your weight, aren't you? So what will you have? Maybe you'll go for the single portion of quiche lorraine to start.

'Pastry is a high-calorie choice.'

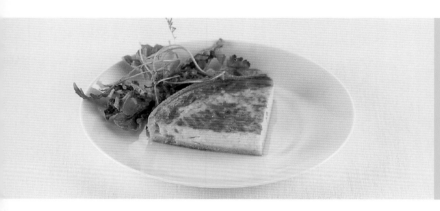

slice of quiche lorraine (200g)

600 calories

Or perhaps you'll go for the piece of tarte tatin for dessert. Beware – either one of these choices alone contains over 500 calories.

or

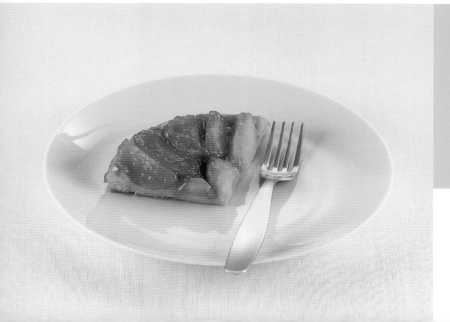

tarte tatin (150g)

530 calories

VS

On the other hand, perhaps you would prefer two courses for fewer calories? For example, you could have this main course of grilled salmon with green beans and couscous, followed by a delicious poached pear. The next time you are struggling over the menu at a restaurant, keep these pictures in mind.

'You don't have to forego a starter or a dessert to keep your calorie intake down.'

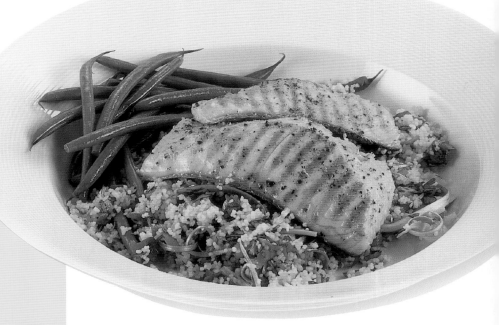

grilled salmon (100g)
210 calories **+**
green beans (50g)
50 calories **+**
couscous (100g)
100 calories **+**
pear poached in red wine
100 calories
_____

460 calories

APÉRITIF OR DINNER?

Care for a drink before dinner? And perhaps a few peanuts while you're sipping your cool drink?

Picture this: the snack and apéritif shown below contain far more calories than the full meal on the right. Have the soup, scallops, vegetables, salad, roll and dessert, and you still won't match the calorie count of the drink and nuts. Even if you add a glass of wine to your meal, the calorie count is less. Surprised?

'That deceptively small bowl of peanuts and the refreshing, long drink may well contain a calorie count bigger than your meal.'

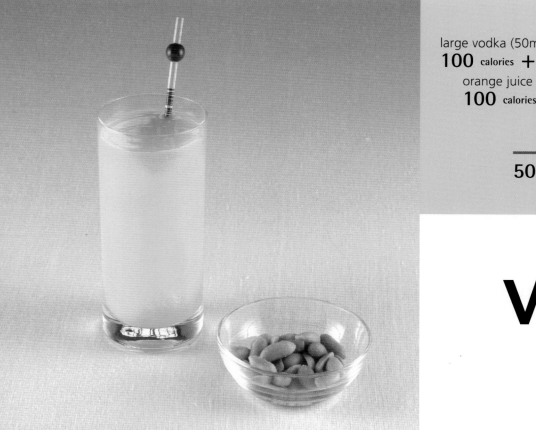

large vodka (50ml)
100 calories **+**
orange juice (200ml)
100 calories **+**
peanuts (50g)
300 calories
___
500 calories

VS

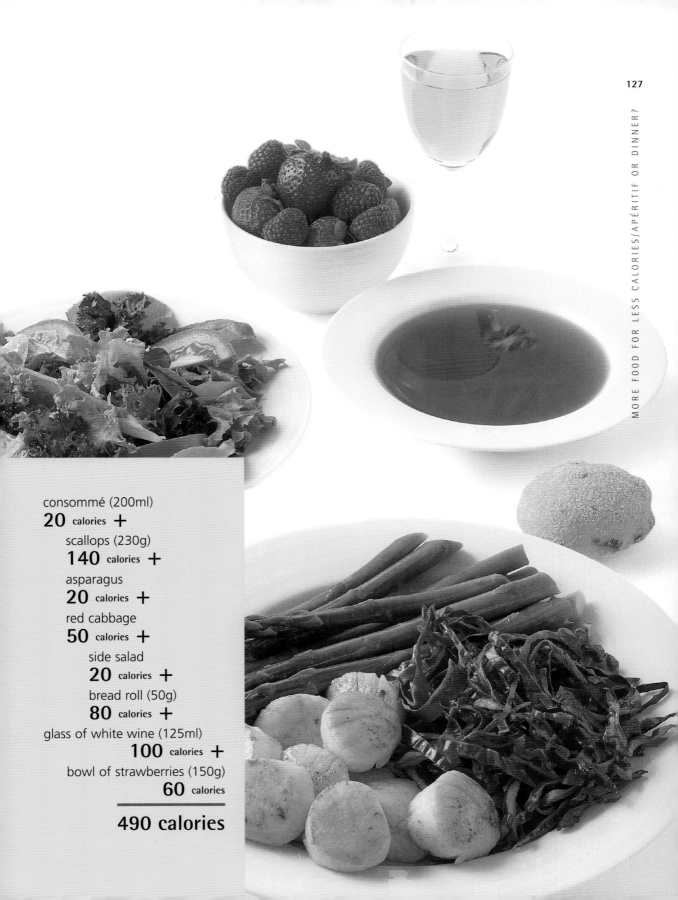

consommé (200ml)
20 calories **+**
scallops (230g)
140 calories **+**
asparagus
20 calories **+**
red cabbage
50 calories **+**
side salad
20 calories **+**
bread roll (50g)
80 calories **+**
glass of white wine (125ml)
100 calories **+**
bowl of strawberries (150g)
60 calories
_____
490 calories

COFFEE

When you're in a café, it's tempting to choose the café latte instead of the standard filter coffee. But just look at the calorie counts. A large latte – even with skimmed milk and no sugar – contains 180 calories. Meanwhile, a filter coffee with milk and two biscuits contains only 130 calories. Next time, you might think twice!

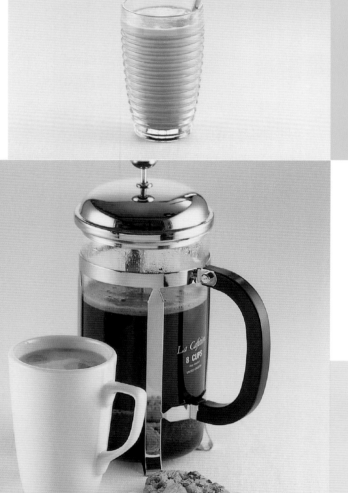

skimmed-milk
café latte (500ml)

180 calories

VS

coffee (500ml) with a
drop of full-cream milk
30 calories
+
2 chocolate chip biscuits
(14g each)
100 calories

130 calories

VALENTINE

Almost criminally delicious, chocolate truffles are also pretty much off the charts, calorie-wise. So. . .what about something else for Valentine's day? Consider offering just a taste or two of truffles and satisfying your beloved's chocolate craving with romantic, chocolate-dipped strawberries instead.

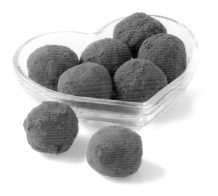

8 chocolate truffles
_____
560 calories

VS

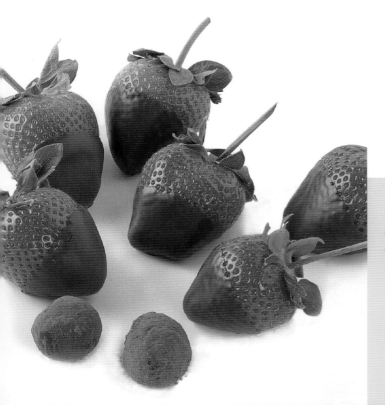

6 strawberries
dipped in chocolate
180 calories

+

2 chocolate truffles
140 calories
_____
320 calories

SWEET TOOTH

This little slice of tiramisu doesn't look like much. And although it may be just the thing for your sweet tooth, it might leave you feeling as if you could have done with a little more.

'Even though the portion of tiramisu is quite small, looks can be deceiving – it contains 500 calories, making it a high-calorie option.'

Looking at the picture on the right should give you something to consider. For the same number of calories as this little slice of tiramisu, you could have a delicious and nutritious selection of fresh fruit, served with frozen yoghurt and biscuits.

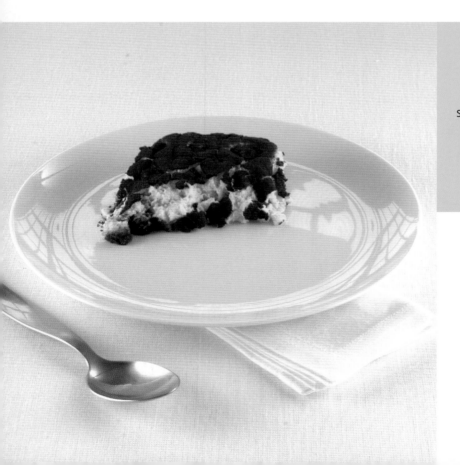

slice of tiramisu (150g)

500 calories

VS

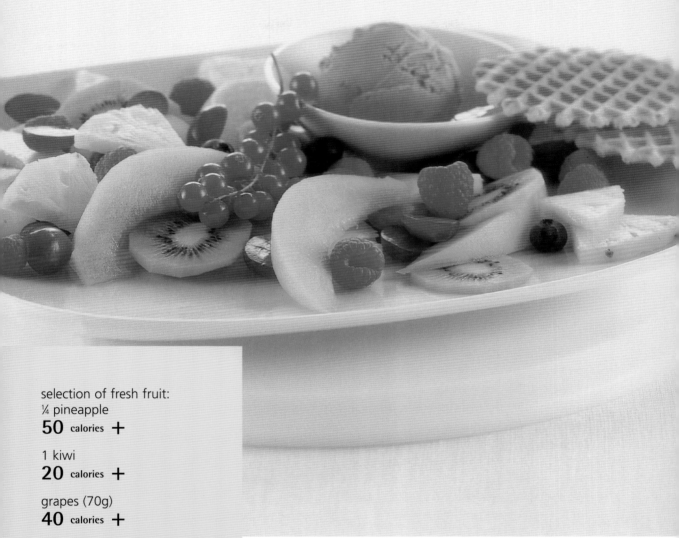

selection of fresh fruit:
¼ pineapple
50 calories **+**

1 kiwi
20 calories **+**

grapes (70g)
40 calories **+**

mixed berries (70g)
20 calories **+**

¼ melon
20 calories **+**

scoop of frozen yoghurt
80 calories **+**

2 biscuits
70 calories
───────────────
300 calories

'This luxurious fruit platter, with all the trimmings, would satisfy anyone's cravings for something sweet.'

SHOPPING LOW-CALORIE

When you begin to change your relationship with food, you'll find yourself making more low-calorie choices almost automatically. But you'll also change your relationship with food shopping. Whether you're a gourmet chef or someone who barely knows how to switch an oven on, you'll want to have a new set of ingredients in the cupboard. By stocking up on the staples of a low-calorie life, you take responsibility for the weight-control choice before you even sit down to a meal. Whenever you reach into the cupboard or pull something out of the freezer, you have already assured yourself of getting a low-calorie option.

ARE PACKAGED FOODS BAD?

I meet many people who, in their yearning for all things natural, have come to distrust processed foods. But it's worth reminding ourselves that most of the chemicals used in food are only there to prevent spoilage and to improve flavour and texture. I don't have anything against canned, packaged or frozen foods. True, you may prefer the taste of fresh foods. But you don't have to avoid packaged foods out of fear of chemical preservatives and other additives.

As for sodium – yes, for some people, there are medical reasons to limit sodium intake. (If you think a low-sodium diet might be necessary for you, speak to your doctor.) But unless you have such a medical condition, there's no reason to avoid sodium. It's simply not an issue as far as fat loss is concerned.

Another misconception is that canning, packaging and freezing remove essential nutrients from food. It is true that a very small amount of nutrients is lost in the process, but certainly not enough to keep you from using processed foods.

As for the freezing process, keep in mind that frozen food is usually of the highest quality. You're getting food that has been frozen at the peak of freshness. You lose nothing, nutrition-wise, when you eat frozen foods, and you gain all the advantages of variety, taste and convenience.

Let's consider a couple of examples. A tin of kidney beans offers a wonderful source of protein along with nutrients, such as folate, fibre, magnesium, iron, copper and potassium. When you open a tin of beans, you get all those advantages without having to go to the bother of soaking and cooking raw beans to make them edible.

Or how about your favourite brand and flavour of vegetable soup? Eating that soup can be a great way to take in vegetables. It's a meal in itself, satisfying and filling as well as tasty and good for you.

In fact, the technologies for preserving food have brought enormous benefits. Wherever we live, we can enjoy fruit and vegetables all year round – tomatoes in December, berries in February. We can buy a supply of groceries that will last for days – and some will stay good for weeks or months. We can cook a whole meal just by boiling water or popping a frozen dinner in the oven.

For anyone making low-calorie choices over a lifetime, the variety and convenience of preserved foods can make a big difference in preventing boredom. And when you prevent boredom, you ensure that you don't end up with that deprived feeling. Don't avoid such foods – embrace them!

LABEL LINGO

Food nutrition labels are a great information source. They're the 'study guide' to a lot of the foods that you're eating, and you'll find them on most food packages these days. But what can you do with the label information?

Knowing what it says on the nutrition information label isn't much good by itself. That's especially the case for people on my programme, because Food Awareness Training does not entail calorie-counting, portion-weighing or nutrient-measuring.

There's no magic number of calories you should or should not eat every day, and no special serving size that will enable you to lose weight. I won't even tell you to eat a certain combination of nutrients that will produce the desired results.

On the other hand, this information is worth knowing. By reading the nutrition information label carefully, you can quickly learn how much of certain nutrients the food contains – paying particular attention to the 'bad guys' such as saturated fat.

To get the most from a food label, you have to read it correctly. Start with the serving size. It's the basis for all the other facts and figures on the label.

Once you've read the serving size, take a moment to think about what you really eat, and compare that to the serving size described on the label. On a jar of olives, the label might indicate that three olives is the serving size, but if you usually eat six, you need to double the calories and all other nutritional figures to find out what you're actually getting when you eat those half-dozen olives.

Government regulations on what information is compulsory on food labelling vary from country to country. In some cases, only the energy value, amount of protein, carbohydrate and fat per 100g or 100ml need be given; for others, the amounts of saturated fat, sugar, dietary fibre and sodium is also required.

If a claim is made about the food – for example, that it is low-fat or contains certain vitamins or minerals – the quantities of these must also be included on the label.

The following definitions apply to the use of certain claims on food packaging:
• A low-calorie food should have 40 calories (167kJ) or less per serving. A low-calorie soft drink must have 10 cal (42 kJ) or less per 100ml.
• A low-fat food should have 3g or less of fat per 100g or 100ml.
• A food that has low saturated fat contains 1.5 g or less of saturated fat per 100g or 100ml.
• A low-sodium food should have 40mg or less of sodium per 100g or 100ml.
• A reduced-energy food should have no more than three quarters of the energy value of a comparable food.

However, these guidelines are only recommendations rather than law in many countries. Your best bet is to look at the label, compare it with other foods, and work out for yourself whether it is a good choice or not.

Knowledge beats ignorance every time. Understanding the data on the label makes you a more informed food shopper and a more thoughtful eater. That's reason enough to browse the nutrition labels when you're making your selections at the supermarket.

READ BEFORE YOU BUY

Caveat emptor! Let the buyer beware! Not everything written on a package means what it says – or says what it means.

Advertising slogans are aimed at selling the product. Few rules apply. Usually, the ads and slogans are in much larger type and more prominently displayed than the food label. So you might be inclined to believe what's printed in the biggest, boldest type. Furthermore, these claims may not be covered by government regulations.

Consider the kind of slogans that are most likely to lure you to the shelves. No cholesterol! proclaims the brightly coloured packet of crisps. Of course, no crisps would have cholesterol, since cholesterol isn't in any food that comes from a vegetable. But those crisps are likely to have hydrogenated fats and lots of calories from fat.

What about sugar-free? It's true that sugar-free sweets probably have no sugar, but what about other sweeteners? The sweets might contain honey, corn syrup, fructose, sorbitol or mannitol. To find out, you'll need to check the small print on the ingredients list. Often, the sugar-free sweets have the same number of calories as 'real' sweets. So why go for the sugar-free? From the all-important vantage point of taste and avoiding feelings of deprivation, you're much better off eating the real thing.

MIND-BOGGLING CLAIMS

Some advertising tactics can be misleading without even trying very hard. One of my favourites is the snack-pack of chocolate-covered raisins advertising '70 per cent less fat'. Look more closely, and you'll see that the packet contains 480 calories. At that rate, you're better off eating a solid chocolate bar. From that, you get about 260 calories.

Apple crisps are another good example. You might think these crisps are simply the shrivelled-up version of the fruit on the tree – an impression that's often reinforced by offering the apple crisps in the health foods or organic aisle. After all, the claim on the bag is '30 per cent less fat than potato crisps'.

But apple chips are a far cry from fresh apples, which are not only easy to eat but also free of added sugar and fat. The crisps have

---

FISHING FOR CUSTOMERS

There's a reason the lettering on that packet is yellow. Yellow is a proven attention-getter. It's the colour the brain processes fastest. So say the researchers who have done extensive studies of colours on mood, attitude and buying habits.

And there's another thing about yellow. It's happy. So if you see a food that's packaged in a bright yellow box – or it's wearing a bright yellow banner – you know why. Cheerful shoppers are more likely to happily buy it.

This is all part of the subtle art of marketing, of course. Experts in consumer research have studied our responses to colours in detail, and they package accordingly. Here's what the findings tell them about our responses:

Red is a colour that increases blood pressure and stimulates appetite.

Green suggests food products that are environmentally sound and probably healthy.

Orange is easy to find. And people find it easier to pay for orange-coloured packaging, experts say.

White means pure, and it also means low in calories.

Brown is simply a rich background colour. (It's unlikely you'll find it at the forefront of any supermarket packaging.)

Blue means fun.

Check out these colours the next time you're in the supermarket. It will help you be aware of what foods, in which packages, are luring you towards them. And why.

added sugar and hydrogenated fat, and they deliver up to 140 calories per serving.

The word 'natural' is nothing more than a marketing tool

I think my favourite marketing claim, however, is the use of the word 'natural'. I'm afraid it can mean just about anything the advertising department wants it to mean. True, many natural foods are healthy and nutritious. A fresh apple, for instance, is full of bountiful nutrients. But what's labelled as natural is not necessarily good for us.

After all, sugar is natural. Cholesterol is natural. Saturated fats are natural. So are tobacco and alcohol. And there's no reason to think that a food made from 'natural ingredients' is the best choice for you when you're watching your weight. A 'naturally sweetened' beverage or biscuit has the same number of calories as a drink or biscuit made with refined sugar.

THE MEANING OF MORE

While we're on the subject of labels and advertising, I might as well bring up one more supermarket trick that can easily get in the way of your weight-control objectives: inducements to buy more. If an item is marked 'two for one' why not just pick up two? You'll save money, and that seems like a sensible bargain. After all, you can always buy two packets of muffins and freeze one. But maybe you don't need that second lot gathering freezer burn, just waiting for you to eat them. You're not getting any bargain at all if you're filling your cupboards with unwanted goods.

REMOVE TEMPTATION

There's no dark conspiracy in this marketing. Food manufacturers hope you will eat more because they want you to buy more. Simple.

Be aware of the inducements used to influence your buying

But be aware of what many studies have shown: you will eat more when there's more to eat. If you buy the family-size packet of crisps, you'll eat more crisps than you would have if you'd just bought the snack size. One recent study showed that people eat as much as 50 per cent more of 'hedonistic foods' — popcorn, crisps, sweets — when they come in bigger packages.

The lesson from all this? Read the label and understand what you're reading. If you're a thoughtful food shopper, you have a better chance of being a thoughtful eater.

PSYCH-OUT LAYOUTS

There is method to the apparent madness of supermarket layouts. First, by dispersing staples all over the place, you are forced to walk past all sorts of attractively packaged and magnificently displayed food products before you get to the food you came for.

Food that's displayed at the end of an aisle is not necessarily a bargain, even though that end-of-the-aisle rack may look like a special offer. Managers know that people notice those displays more than products on the rest of the shelves. So products with the highest mark-up are carefully positioned to catch your eye.

Shelf level counts, too. The first things you see are products at your eye level. For children, eye level is lower. Notice where the children's sweets and snacks are located – at just about your waist level, where the kids will be transfixed by the sight of them.

WHAT TO BUY

Nearly all of us have access to supermarkets. Quality and size vary, but every supermarket – from one of the huge national chains to a smaller, regional establishment – offers some variety of choice. If you live in a large metropolitan area with speciality shops and health food stores, so much the better.

> ## Grab anything that adds flavour or variety to your food

Let's have a quick look at some of your selections. The nucleus of your supermarket tours will be what I call the Anytime List that you'll find on page 138. This list has foods to keep on hand to eat at any time, either as a snack or as part of a meal, such as vegetables, fruit and the lowest-calorie frozen desserts and sweets available. Make these the core of your eating, and you stand a superb chance of being thin for life.

Load your shopping cart with low-fat condiments of every variety to give your food extra flavour. Enjoying your food is essential for both weight loss and a lifetime of weight control. Then head for the frozen food aisle. If you're the type of person who needs a quick meal occasionally, you may wish to toss a few frozen low-calorie complete meals into your shopping trolley, along with a generous supply of frozen vegetables and fruit. Above all, don't forget frozen seafood.

Also stock up on a good range of drinks that suit your tastes. There is a profusion of low-calorie hot chocolates available. Most range from 20 to 50 calories per packet (it's best to avoid hot beverages that carry more than that). Check the labels – avoid drinks labelled 'naturally sweetened' or 'fruit-juice sweetened', since they tend to be full of calories.

Once your cabinets and freezer are stuffed with the basics, going shopping becomes pretty much a matter of buying the fresh foods that complete the meal.

FRUIT AND VEG

Just about everything in the fresh produce section offers the fewest number of calories – and the biggest fibre punch – relative to the quantity of food you eat. The more you make fresh vegetables the basis of your diet, the thinner and healthier you will be.

If your idea of vegetables is limited to a salad with iceberg lettuce or the spinach your mother made you eat as a child, think again. Now, within our reach is food that's imported from all over the world.

If you see the less-than-familiar in your produce aisle, why not take the opportunity to try a new taste sensation? Try the daikon radish from Japan – superb in salads, dressings and soups. Try yams from Africa – good in soups or casseroles. Or add pak choi from China to stir-fries: its leaves have a crisp texture and mild taste.

Of course, it's fine to stick with the old standbys if you prefer. Green beans, yellow peppers, carrots, aubergine, peas, sprouts, mushrooms, cabbage, onions, broccoli, parsnip, cucumber, watercress. . . The range of tastes is staggering.

> ## The global market offers many new taste opportunities

Like vegetables, fruit is high in fibre, rich in nutrients and low in calories. And like vegetables, it has gone global. In fact, the names of the most nutritionally dense fruit may surprise you. They are, in order, kiwi fruit, papaya, mango and orange. Kiwi is

IN PRAISE OF PULSES

Pulses offer the person trying to lose weight a double dose of benefits. First, they are low in fat and packed with nutrients: fibre, phytochemicals, folate, protein, magnesium, potassium, zinc, copper, iron and vitamins.

Second, the potential they offer for culinary creativity is as staggering as their variety. From Cuban black beans and rice to Indian daal (lentils), from Israeli hummus (chickpeas) to Egyptian ful medames (broad beans), you can eat a different dish virtually every night of the week.

loaded with vitamin C – about twice as much, in fact, as an orange. It also has hearty amounts of potassium and magnesium. Other tropicals, such as guava and kumquat, are also high in fibre and rich in nutrients.

Another option is dried fruit. Unsweetened apricots, figs, dates and pears have no more calories when they're dried than they did when they were freshly picked. (But you have to check the labels – dried pineapple and papaya usually contain a lot of sugar and more calories than the fresh fruit. And stay away from banana chips – they're not simply dried, they're fried in fat.)

YES, THEY'RE GOOD FOR YOU

Generally, however, my recommendation for fruit and vegetables is simple: the more the merrier. Nothing is better for weight control or for your health. All vegetables and fruit are full of vitamins, minerals and phytochemicals that keep us healthy and help stave off disease.

The high fibre content is particularly helpful for weight control. High-fibre foods can take the edge off appetite. Fibre is not digested or absorbed – it takes up space in the intestine, thus contributing to a sense of satiety. So eating a lot of vegetables and fruit keeps calorie intake low and reduces hunger.

GO WITH THE GRAIN

Wholegrain breads, pastas, cereals and crackers all have excellent nutritional benefits. They are good carriers of iron, fibre and the B-complex vitamins. From the point of view of weight control, they're also very satisfying and filling – good 'comfort foods'.

But they also tend to be high in carbohydrate calories. My recommendation is to look at the starches as a lower-priority food – far below vegetables, fruit, pulses and seafood in the hierarchy of best choices.

In fact, I recommend that you look for the light breads now offered in some stores. These have around 40 to 45 calories per slice. What's more, the slices are regular-size, not those wafer-thin slivers that turn to mush at the first touch of tuna salad.

As for breakfast cereals, try to find one that's a good fibre buy for the calories. The best choices are usually the bran-based ones.

You may also want to have some refined grain products such as white rice, couscous, pasta, polenta and the like – but enjoy them in moderation. Have a small bowl of linguine, for instance, or a light helping of rice. Of course, you can add as many vegetables as you like.

DR SHAPIRO'S ANYTIME LIST

The following foods are the best bets for any time of year. If you have these foods at the ready, they'll be the first that you reach for when you're hungry. So here's my prescription for the foods that you should keep on hand.

VEGETABLES
All kinds of vegetables – raw, cooked, fresh, frozen, tinned or in soups.

FRUIT
All fruit – raw or cooked, fresh, frozen or tinned. (Avoid any packaged fruit with added sugar.)

DRINKS
Help yourself to any low-calorie drinks. Ones to keep in stock include:

Coffees and teas Including fruit and herbal teas and iced tea and coffee
Diet fizzy drinks Any preference of flavours
Instant hot chocolate Look for mixes that have 20 to 50 calories per serving. Avoid cocoa mixes that have 60 calories or more
Milkshake mixes You want the kinds that have 70 or fewer calories per serving

FROZEN DESSERTS
All kinds of fat-free frozen yoghurt, sorbet or ice lollies are good to have in your freezer. When selecting brands, be sure to keep an eye on the calories.

SWEETS
Chewing gum
Hard-boiled sweets Such as lollipops, rock, humbugs and butterscotch

CONDIMENTS AND SEASONINGS
All the flavourful ingredients listed below are low-calorie. Use them creatively to spice up your vegetable courses, treats and snacks.

Oil-free or low-calorie salad dressings
Fat-free or low-fat mayonnaise, low-fat créme fraîche
Fat-free yoghurt Natural or artificially sweetened
Mustards Dijon and other kinds
Tomato Purée, passata, tomato juice
Lemon or lime juice
Oil sprays In butter or olive-oil flavours
Vinegars Balsamic, cider, tarragon, wine or other flavours
Sauces Barbecue, chutney, ketchup, relish, salsa, soy, tamari, Worcestershire, hoisin, horseradish, miso, black bean and oyster
Onion Fresh, flakes or powder
Garlic Fresh, purée, flakes or powder
Herbs All kinds, including basil, bay leaves, chives, dill, oregano, rosemary, sage, tarragon and thyme
Spices All kinds, including allspice, cinnamon, cloves, coriander, cumin, curry powder, ginger, nutmeg, paprika and pepper
Extracts Including almond, coconut, peppermint and vanilla
Cocoa powder
Stock cubes

DAIRY DO'S AND DON'TS

In the dairy aisle, you may hear the echo of your mother's voice. Remember when you were a child and she kept telling you, 'Milk is good for you'? Well, it turns out this may not be the case. Recent research has found evidence that milk and other dairy products may contribute to breast cancer, ovarian cancer, even diabetes – and substituting low-fat dairy products will not eliminate these risks.

In addition to posing these health risks, milk may also be less helpful in preventing bone loss than we once thought. Since dairy products are high in calcium, doctors long assumed that dairy products could help prevent osteoporosis. New evidence contradicts this assumption: animal protein (including dairy) actually stimulates the loss of calcium through the kidneys, which will accelerate the pace of osteoporosis.

Another issue with dairy products is their fat content. Unless they're fat-free (like skimmed milk), dairy products contain highly saturated fat: the very worst kind. However, many dairy products, such as milk, yoghurt and cheese, come in low-fat versions. This can make a significant difference. Low-fat Cheddar cheese might have 250 calories per 100 grams, while ordinary Cheddar has almost double that amount – about 430 calories per 100 grams. Unfortunately, many low-fat dairy products leave something to be desired in the flavour and texture department.

If you choose to eat dairy and think you can dodge the fat issue, read the labels carefully. Some low-fat cheese is really just lower-fat. The range can be confusing. One reduced-fat cheese might offer as little as 40 calories and 6 grams of fat per 100 grams. Another, reduced-fat cheese might have 270 calories and 24 grams of fat per 100 grams – which puts it in the range of a really good Brie.

GO FISH!

Because fish carry a considerable amount of muscle on their spindly little skeletons, they are an exceptionally good source of complete protein. Fish supplies a wealth of iron and other minerals. You can eat fish any way you like – filleted, skinned, fresh, smoked, frozen or canned. Or help yourself to sushi.

In addition, fish is rich in vitamins. And it contains essential fatty acids – like omega-3s and omega-6s – that your body requires for turning food into energy (the process of metabolism). In fact, fish are the only animals that carry these good kinds of fat. And – as a rule – the richer the fish, the more good fat there is.

To top off all these benefits, fish is low in calories. So, for purposes of weight control, it's almost a perfect food.

SUGAR SURPRISES

You know there's sugar in foods such as chocolate bars and cola. But did you ever suspect that orange juice, apple sauce and most flavoured yoghurts also have sugar? Lots of it, in fact.

In addition to the sugar that occurs naturally in these foods, much more may be added. A glass of one brand of orange juice drink, for example, contains 22 grams of sugar – double the amount that occurs naturally in an orange. A pot of vanilla low-fat yoghurt with raspberries may have as much as 51 grams of sugar.

The whole story may not be apparent from the label. Since sugar comes in many forms, check the label for corn syrup, fructose, honey, molasses, even fruit juice concentrate.

While it's perfectly true that there are many high-sugar, low-calorie foods that can be included in a weight-loss programme – think of sorbets or hard-boiled sweets, for example – you should beware of any foods that contain hidden sugar calories.

MEET THE MEATS AND POULTRY

I am not going to lecture you on the benefits of a vegetarian diet. But it is certainly a very healthy way to eat, and I am going to try to acquaint you with tasty meat substitutes.

An increasingly wide range of soya products is available today to replace foods like sausages, burgers, ham and even bacon. We can also get soya milk, tofu, tempeh, miso and, of course, soy sauce. In fact, if you're in search of soya, you can find a food fit for almost any taste and any occasion. Tried any recently? Soya products are surprisingly tasty. Even the leanest meat or poultry cannot compete with these products in terms of low calories and health benefits.

In general, there are better sources of protein and iron than you'll find in red meat and poultry. So eat sparingly. If and when you do eat meat, look for particularly lean cuts. Skinless poultry is somewhat better for you than red meat because it's lower in fat, but I have trouble giving wholehearted endorsement to chicken because it has a high concentration of certain cancer-causing substances. Again, soya replacements make sense.

WHY SOYA SO OFTEN?

As you can probably tell, I'm a great fan of soya products for everyone – but especially for anyone trying to lose weight. There are a number of reasons for my enthusiasm.

In a study that included people from 59 different countries, researchers showed that the more soya people ate, the lower the rate of fatal prostate cancer. Soya was four times more likely to prevent prostate cancer than any other ingredient in the diet.

In Asian countries where soya has long been a culinary staple, the incidence of breast and prostate cancer is far below that of

SOME PROBLEMS WITH MEAT

We've long known that undercooked meat can pose a threat to your health. It can contain dangerous *E. coli* bacteria, or an aggressive strain of salmonella bacteria that is resistant to antibiotics.

On top of that, now comes news that cooked meat can also cause problems. Certain carcinogens generated by the process of heating meat can lead to colon cancer and breast cancer. Studies in both Finland and the United States confirm that it's these carcinogens rather than the fat content in meat that create a higher risk of breast cancer. Other studies have shown that the risk of colorectal cancer is greater in people who eat a substantial amount of meat, and that men who make meat their main dish five or six times a week are 2.5 times more likely to get prostate cancer than men who eat little or no meat.

Many people assumed that these carcinogens were found only in red meat. Now there's evidence that chicken may carry the same risk – perhaps even higher. Whether you grill, fry or barbecue the chicken, the levels climb the longer it's cooked.

In general, the health-care costs for people who eat meat are far higher than the medical costs for vegetarians or even semi-vegetarians. That's something to chew on.

Western countries. Recent studies in the United States, Japan and China confirm that even one serving of soya per day can halve the risk of colon, rectal, lung and breast cancer. It may also help protect against osteoporosis.

In addition to its other virtues, soya packs a sensational nutritional wallop. As a protein source, it is comparable to meat and eggs. It also contains iron, B vitamins, calcium and zinc. With soya, you'll get a power-packed supply of good health. And nearly all soya foods that are considered 'substitutes' have fewer calories than the foods or ingredients they're replacing.

THE GOURMET IN YOUR SOUL

This is not a cookbook, and I am not a chef. I am far more at home in my surgery than in the kitchen. But there are some tips on food preparation that make sense even to me.

Firstly, grill, steam, bake or poach your food; don't fry it. Frying by definition is a fat-adding, high-calorie cooking process. It's bad for your health and for your waistline. (Notice how frequently the two go together!)

Secondly, open the bottle. Open up the Worcestershire sauce or hoisin or salsa and use the contents liberally. Brush your own marinade over vegetables before putting them on the grill. Spice up a tomato sauce with Tabasco and lemon juice instead of using just plain old ketchup on your soya burger. In short, be creative. You may discover a superb new dish, a hidden talent for creating chutneys or a special liking for sprouts. The point is to not feel deprived, to not be bored. With a cupboard and freezer stocked with the vast array of choices on the Anytime List, you'll be able to prepare food that's tasty as well as low-calorie and healthy. Eating is a pleasure as well as a necessity.

AN EATING OUT CHECK LIST

If you're on a diet, few things are more terrifying than dining out at a restaurant. Either you're afraid you won't be able to resist the temptation of delicious foods and will stray from the diet, or you're worried that if you favour the dieter's typical meal of steamed fish and salad – no dressing, please – everyone will know you're dieting. There will follow the inevitable expressions of surprise, support, dismissal, encouragement or interest – all of which you'd rather live without.

The alternative, of course, is to stay at home. But life goes on, and part of life is going out to restaurants. And so it should be. One of life's pleasures is enjoying the world's vast variety of tastes and traditions and innovations in eating, without having to prepare the food or clean up afterwards. Of course you're going to dine out. The issue for the weight-conscious is dining out without being done in.

Fortunately, menus everywhere offer an array of options. All you have to do is find and choose the low-calorie, healthy option.

1. You're looking for the lowest- or lower-calorie choice. For example, garlic prawns sautéed in butter might be a top choice if they were the only seafood, but would move down the scale of desirability if there are lower-calorie fish dishes on the menu.

2. Consider not just the amount of fat in a dish but the kind of fat as well. A pesto sauce may be high in fat, but derives from vegetable sources – pine nuts and olive oil – which qualify as 'good fats', versus the 'bad' saturated fat from animal sources in a cream sauce.

3. Proteins from fish and shellfish, soya products and pulses are preferable to proteins from meat, poultry and dairy produce.

4. Fruit and vegetables offer the greatest calorie bargain. They also give you the most rewards in terms of needed vitamins, minerals and fibre.

5. Most desserts are high in calories. If part of the reason you're eating out is to splurge, go ahead. But if eating out is something you do all the time, think twice about dessert.

THE EXERCISE COMPONENT

Every health professional in the country advises patients that exercise is important. Every new piece of research confirms it. Every reader of newspapers is aware of it.

Exercise helps prevent disease by strengthening your immune system. It makes you feel better, sleep better, work better. It improves your appearance. It raises your energy level. It even lifts your mood. And, proved beyond all doubt, exercise helps you lose and control weight.

The connection between exercise and weight control is as simple as it is obvious: exercise burns calories. Specifically, exercise builds and strengthens muscles, and muscle cells burn calories more efficiently than fat cells do. And since weight loss is a matter of using up more calories than you take in, exercise is an important part of the weight-loss battle.

But there are other factors as well – some hidden but proven virtues that also play a big role. Exercise can actually decrease appetite. And, just as importantly, exercise can reduce the stress that so often influences appetite.

Whenever you exercise, it's beneficial

In fact, the ultimate equation for weight loss in this book can be summed up pretty simply: lower-calorie food choices plus walking or light home exercise equal weight loss and weight control for life.

Research increasingly confirms that even short bouts of exercise, spaced intermittently throughout the day, enhance your overall fitness and contribute to weight control. A brisk walk up and down stairs, 10 minutes of lifting homemade weights or a quarter of an hour on an exercise bike all provide boosts to your system. And, say researchers, what counts is the total accumulation of exercise in a 24-hour period. In other words, all exercise counts.

STARTING ON THE RIGHT FOOT

If you're starting the weight-loss programme in this book and you're not now involved in regular exercise, it's time to start an exercise programme as well. Together, exercise and healthy, low-calorie food choices can help you control your weight for the rest of your life, and can also help keep you fit, trim and energetic – in short, the picture of health.

Of course, say the word 'exercise' and the picture that inevitably comes to mind is that of the professional athlete. That's not what I expect. It's both unrealistic and unnecessary for you to become Jonathan Edwards launching into the air for the triple jump, or Paula Radcliffe looking like she barely feels the strain as she nears the 10,000 metre mark. Both of these athletes are certainly worthy standards to aim for, but that level of training and fitness isn't what you need to help you with weight loss.

In fact, for the kind of exercise I'm suggesting, you don't need to join a gym or buy fancy equipment. You don't even need to take up a sport. All of those are great ideas, but if you don't particularly like sport, or you don't like the expense and ambience of a health club, or you're not into exercise equipment, you still have lots of opportunities for exercise. In fact, you don't even have to leave the house if you don't want to. There's only one slight challenge: getting enough exercise.

You don't have to change your lifestyle to get more exercise

I want you to approach physical activity with the same awareness with which you're now learning to approach your food choices. The information and the photographs in this book help you understand your low-calorie options among foods. In the same way, with some awareness of your exercise options, you can get in the habit of choosing the energetic, more physically demanding option among available activities.

CHOOSE TO MOVE

The fact is that we live in a sedentary age. Once upon a time, our forebears had to sweat just to live. Eating meant going out on hunting and gathering expeditions every day. To get enough food, our ancestors had to do a significant amount of walking, running and climbing. The necessity for warmth and light meant gathering fuel. This entailed more walking, more gathering, plus the furious activity of rubbing together two sticks – humankind's first exercise equipment.

Of course, driving to the supermarket doesn't involve the same calorific burn as hunting wild boar. And we're paying a price for our indolence. We've also come a long way from the era of our grandparents. They at least had to get up out of their chairs to change the channel on their TVs. Pretty soon, according to researcher James Levine at the Mayo Clinic in Rochester, Minnesota, 'we won't even need to expend the energy to

EXERCISE AND HEART DISEASE

Some recent studies are shedding light on the effects of exercise on triglycerides, a type of fat that contributes to cardiovascular disease. It has long been suspected that the influx of these fats into the bloodstream after eating – especially after heavy eating – actually damages blood vessels. The more rapidly the triglycerides can be cleared out of the blood, therefore, the lower the risk of heart disease.

Exercise, it has now been shown, increases the enzyme in the body that breaks down triglycerides and thus gets them out of the bloodstream fast.

In one study conducted in England, researchers measured the triglyceride levels among two groups of women both before and after they walked. The first group was asked to walk at a moderate pace for 1 hour while the second group walked for 2 hours. The next day, all the women were fed a high-fat meal. Those who had walked for 1 hour showed a 12 per cent lower trigylceride level, while the 2-hour walkers reduced their post-meal triglyceride levels by 23 per cent.

The equation is simple: more walking equals faster breakdown of triglycerides, which equals lower coronary risk.

push a button. We'll just say "bring me the food" and computers will operate on voice recognition. We'll become immobile blobs.'

Organised, regular physical activity can help avoid the 'immobile blob' fate. But the real antidote is not strenuous effort. Rather, it's getting more physical activity into our lifestyles. In other words: move, and make movement a part of just about everything you do.

Choosing the stairs instead of the lift makes a big difference

As with food, a physically active lifestyle is all about awareness and choice. It means parking as far as possible from the supermarket and walking the rest of the way. It means taking the stairs whenever possible. It means mowing or raking the lawn yourself instead of paying the boy down the street to do it. It means walking to the shop to get the morning paper instead of having it delivered.

I'll also recommend some exercises you can do easily, in your own home, to extend and expand the benefits of physical activity for weight loss. As with changing your relationship with food, the change in your relationship with physical activity is not aimed at overturning your lifestyle. The idea instead is to make exercise an integral part of what you do every day. Some form of exercise can become as much a habit as low-calorie food decisions.

When you are automatically mindful of both your food choices and your activity choices – when your routine consists of walking to the high street to get a low-calorie lunch and then walking back – you'll be set to control your weight for life.

EXERCISE BASICS

The experts divide exercise into three components: aerobics, strength training and flexibility.

Aerobic exercise – walking, jogging, dancing, cycling, even climbing the stairs – uses your large muscle groups and works your heart, lungs and circulatory system. By definition, aerobic exercise releases energy through the use of oxygen; it requires endurance rather than power.

Strength training or weight-bearing exercise builds muscle tissue, and bigger muscles burn more calories. What's more, since we lose muscle mass as we age – about 30 per cent of our total number of muscle cells between ages 20 and 70 – anything that counteracts that loss also counteracts the

FLEXING THROUGH TRAFFIC

Cut the stress of your car journey and burn calories at the same time. While waiting at the lights or while you're stuck in a traffic jam, try these exercises.
■ Press your lower back into the seat and tighten your abdominal muscles for a few seconds. Work your 'glutes' – that is, squeeze your buttocks together.
■ Stretch your neck down towards your left shoulder, then towards your right.
■ Squeeze the steering wheel. Release. Squeeze again.
■ Set your hands at 9 o'clock and 3 o'clock on the steering wheel. Press your elbows together.
■ Lift both shoulders. Hold. Then release.
■ Leaning forwards in your seat, press your shoulders back, trying to make your shoulder blades touch.
■ Move your head forwards and from side to side.
■ Tighten every muscle in your body. Relax. These are also great exercises if you're in an aeroplane!

effects of ageing. And despite the name, strength training isn't just about lifting weights. Any activity in which your muscles work against resistance counts. That includes everything from playing football to learning the tango.

Finally, flexibility exercising – stretching – not only helps 'lubricate' the body for effective exercise and for injury prevention, but it also improves balance and coordination while enhancing your physical performance. Think of your muscles as springs. If they're short and tight, they have little room for motion when they're contracted. But if you stretch your muscles – slowly, easily, deliberately – they'll respond with power. Muscles that are more flexible and powerful also allow you a wider range of motion. That can make quite a difference as

you get older. A regular programme of stretching can help reduce some of the most immobilising effects of ageing.

In addition, a slow, focused stretching routine is a great relaxation technique. It reduces anxiety along with muscle tension and lowers blood pressure along with your breathing rate.

Not surprisingly, the best exercise programme includes all three types of movement – aerobics, strength training and flexibility exercises. The perfect workout starts with a simple warm-up – about 5 minutes of gentle movement. Then stretch. After that, do some aerobic and strength-training exercise. Finally, cool down and finish with another stretch at the end. You can do just about all of this in one perfect exercise that I call POW – Plain Old Walking.

STRENGTH TRAINING FOR WEIGHT LOSS

Our metabolisms slow as we age. In fact, it's estimated that with each passing decade, the body needs 100 fewer calories per day. This would be an argument for eating fewer calories the older we get. But there's another way to compensate for the reduced calorie needs that accompany ageing. Since exercise speeds metabolism, we'll burn more calories if we get more intense physical activity.

As we get older, however, we probably have to strategise if we want to increase exercise and burn calories. After all, we're inclined to 'slow down' rather than 'speed up' as we get older – aren't we?

So what's the answer? How can we get more of that 'burn' going? One solution is strength training. By counteracting muscle

loss, strength training helps increase metabolism – by as much as 10 to 15 per cent by some estimates. Just two or three strength-training sessions a week can help. And strength training is not weight lifting. You're not going for a body-builder's physique. It just means lifting weights in a very slow, controlled way to build muscle tone and burn calories.

Along with its other benefits, strength training can help you feel more youthful. While nothing can actually halt the ageing process and its effects on weight, strength training seems to slow the process and mitigate the effects.

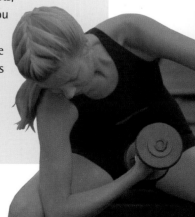

OFF AND WALKING

The perfect exercise is right at your feet. The more we learn about the benefits of walking, the better it gets.

Walking is superb for heart health and for maintaining muscle mass. It is low-impact; it strengthens bones, it doesn't hurt them. Where weight is concerned, you can almost literally 'walk it off', not to mention the fact that walking can give you lean, shapely thighs and buttocks. And, of course, walking will give you rosy cheeks, clear the cobwebs out of your mind and give you deep sleep and, more likely than not, pleasant dreams.

> **Walking improves your coordination, speed and agility**

But there's more. We also know that walking can help prevent cancers of the colon and prostate. It counteracts gall bladder problems. It aids metabolism. It helps prevent osteoporosis. And it has been proven to be an important preventative against adult-onset diabetes – type 2 diabetes. A recent study by the American National Institutes of Health showed that brisk walking helped keep diabetes at bay and/or minimised its effects. The study covered 1500 people, and the results held true whether the study subjects had the disease, were predisposed to it or were free of it. All it took was a brisk, half-hour walk several days a week.

We're also learning that walking for exercise need not mean a lengthy 'power walk' or an all-day hike. Even brief, intermittent walks – say three 10-minute walks interspersed throughout the day – can make an enormous difference to your overall health and to your weight-control efforts.

For a while, it was popular to carry hand weights or strap on ankle weights to enhance calorie burn and strength building. But I don't advise it. Carrying weights when you walk for exercise adds little in the way of aerobic intensity and may actually alter your gait, put pressure on your neck and shoulders and even make you injury-prone. For more aerobic intensity, walk uphill, quicken your pace or walk a greater distance.

TAKING IT IN YOUR STRIDE

How can you get started? Just lace up a pair of comfortable, sturdy shoes, open the door, step outside and go. You don't need special equipment for walking; you can do it anywhere; you can do it alone or with company, and the neighbours won't think you're loopy when they see you treading briskly past their front windows. After all, you're just out for a walk. Best of all, this is

TABLE TENNIS, ANYONE?

The only racket and ball game you can play in the house, table tennis is a highly effective calorie-burner, blitzing about 300 calories an hour. That's equivalent to a brisk walk, but table tennis also exercises the playing arm in addition to the heart and legs. What's more it's fun, and the competitive element keeps your interest up – you can even organise family tournaments. You'll have done hours of exercise before you know it!

an exercise you already know how to do. As with any exercise, start slowly at first. Move at a comfortable, easy pace for at least the first 10 minutes – or until you feel ready to pick up the pace.

If it's cold outside, dress in layers – long underwear (if it's really cold), then a T-shirt and tracksuit bottoms, topped with a sports sweater or jacket. You'll warm up as you go, and you can shed the outer layers – tying the sweater or jacket around your waist.

Count on getting thirsty. Pack a water bottle in a pocket or backpack.

And the rest . . . well, just enjoy it. Swing your arms. Stretch your legs. Loosen your shoulders. Look at the scenery; it changes with the seasons. Hum. Whistle. Sing. When you get back home, stretch your body. Feel how loose and strong you are.

That's all it takes – just going for a walk two or three times a week. If you find yourself getting bored with the walks in your area, drive to another area or into the

Take a personal stereo and listen to your favourite tunes

countryside. Try some other kinds of changes. Alter your pace. Speed up for 2 minutes, then slow down and stroll. Go into long strides, then drop back to a short, quick pace. Change the distance you walk. Or try some hills. Pump your arms on the uphill and keep your knees soft on the downhill.

If it's raining or snowing, or the weather is unpleasantly hot and humid, then drive to the nearest shopping centre. Just before the shops open is a great time to stride through the centre – and you're always guaranteed perfect conditions.

A RISK-REDUCER FOR MEN

A recent study involving 51,000 male health-care professionals has demonstrated that physical activity can lower the risk of benign prostatic hyperplasia, BPH, an enlargement of the prostate gland that causes frequent urination and is particularly common in older men. Walking for 2 to 3 hours per week lowered the risk by 25 per cent – not to mention its benefits to weight loss and overall fitness.

Of course, there's nothing wrong with walking in the rain. It's only water, after all. Just buy some good protective clothing so you don't catch a chill.

THE WORK/WALK OPTIONS

Many people drive or take public transport to work from door to door, but there are ways to introduce some extra steps into your travels.

If you take public transport, you can get off one stop early or a few streets away from work – then walk the rest of the way.

If you drive to work, you may find yourself jostling for the parking space that's nearest to the front door. What about reversing that trend? Park as far away as possible and walk to the office. It will clear your mind for the day ahead as well as help with fitness and weight loss.

Once you're there, can you walk upstairs for that meeting? Or at least walk at a fast pace from office to office?

What do you do on your breaks? If you get an hour for lunch, why not spend 30 minutes on a light meal and the rest on a brisk walk? You can even make yourself popular by offering to run errands for your colleagues – and get the benefit of some exercise on the way.

EXERCISES AT HOME

In addition to walking, there are many exercises you can do at home for minimal cost or none at all. In the same National Institutes of Health study where doctors looked at the effect of walking, they also discovered benefits from simple household chores and activities. Such light 'exercises' as gardening and cleaning the bathroom carry many of the same benefits as walking.

Exercising at home is a great option if you have kids

Apart from routine activities, you can get special benefits from simple weight-lifting exercises. Not only do these exercises build strength, but they can also help sculpt your arm and leg muscles at the same time.

All you need are 1- or 2-kilogram weights. These are available at most sports shops. Alternatively, take a couple of old socks and fill them with dried beans or even with coins. Or fill a pair of empty 1-litre plastic bottles with sand or water.

Another alternative for strength training is the elastic exercise band. You can get these bands for a few pounds in sports shops, and they will typically come with an illustrated booklet on how to use them. The bands have different ranges of resistance, from easy to medium to high. A workout of half a dozen exercises with these bands strengthens and tones virtually every muscle in the body. Furthermore, the bands can travel with you. Just toss them in your briefcase or suitcase when you leave.

HOPS, SKIPS AND JUMPS

Did you ever skip in the school playground as a child? This may be a good time to try it again. It is superb for building cardiovascular endurance, working the upper-body muscles as well as the legs and burning lots and lots of calories. It's also an activity you can do in the dead of winter.

Skipping is not the knee-cracking bone-crusher some people think it is. When you do it right, you're only jumping a little way off the ground, making skipping a fairly low-impact exercise. Plus, all you need is a rope.

GOING IN CYCLES

Did you know that cycling is one of the best forms of exercise you can do? It offers a great workout for the heart and circulatory system. With cycling you burn from 400 to 700 calories an hour. While you're pedalling away, you are strengthening your quadriceps and even your abdominals. Cycling puts little stress on your joints, except your knees. And if you keep the seat high, you can even reduce pressure on your knees.

As for bikes, they range from mountain bikes to racers, and come in all sizes and shapes. Just make sure you get 'fitted' for the right bike at a good cycling shop – and also get a good helmet. Once you're kitted out, cycling is a sport you can do just about anywhere, in just about any season.

DIFFERENT STROKES

Swimming – or any water workout – is the perfect high-aerobic, low-impact exercise. It works the quadriceps, hamstrings, biceps, triceps, abdominals and gluteal muscles while building stamina.

Swimming is often a good alternative exercise for people who have chronic pain.

When you're swimming, there's no jarring or shock to the body. With the water keeping you buoyant and supporting your body weight, there is no pressure on your joints or tendons. What's more, you don't have to know how to swim like an expert – even a workout in the shallow end can be beneficial.

VIDEO GUIDES

If you haven't checked out the health and exercise collection at your local video shop, make sure you have a look. The number and variety of aerobics programme tapes are staggering. Aerobics isn't just jumping on the spot while moving your arms anymore, either. You can find exercise sessions modelled on everything from African dance to martial arts, from disco nights to belly dancing to military boot camp.

If you work shifts, you can still exercise on your own schedule

If you think the same video will eventually become boring (and it might), just turn on the television. Cable networks are brimming with exercise shows.

Stretching and/or yoga videos are also easy to come by. You might also want to have a look in your local library or book shop for books and tapes.

One caution, however. Remember to warm up and stretch before exercising, then cool down and stretch afterwards. Often the warm-ups and stretches are part of the video, but even if they're not, you need them to prevent injury and to get the most benefit out of your exercise.

Static stretching is the safest kind. Do the stretch through the muscle's range of motion until you feel resistance – in the form of tightening or even the first stirrings of discomfort. Hold the stretch at that point for at least 10 seconds, then relax. Never go past the point of pain or discomfort.

YOUR STAIRS ARE YOUR FRIENDS

If you live in a house, you may not realise it but you have a built-in health club. Walk up those stairs. Then walk down; then up again. Increase the number of times you go up and down. Over time, as your confidence grows, you may want to speed up your pace as well. If you live in a block of flats, walk up as many flights as you can; you'll find that the number you can manage comfortably increases as you become more fit.

Even if you live in a bungalow, you can get the same benefit from 'step exercising'. Buy a step from your local sports shop. It may seem like a simple exercise to step up and down from a single step – but if you pace yourself, you'll get all the benefits of stair-climbing.

EXERCISE UNLIMITED

If you want to go beyond these home exercises, you can, of course, choose from among a greater range of activities, including many that are more rigorous. Joining a gym is great – if you go regularly. You can use a variety of exercise equipment designed to exercise different parts of your body, from weight machines to exercise bikes – and you can get advice from specialists at the gym, who can help design an exercise programme especially for you.

Learning to play a sport is wonderful – if you can find team-mates and if you enjoy it. And bringing high-powered equipment into your home, such as treadmills, exercise bikes and the like, can be a big help – if you remember to use the equipment.

Above all, don't be limited by the obvious, traditional exercise activities. There's a world of alternatives out there: interesting activities that are fun, that stretch the mind and soul along with the body, that feel less like working out than like undertaking an adventure and learning a new, fulfilling skill.

You can sign up for one of the many exercise classes available at gyms and sports centres, such as step aerobics and yoga. These classes are also a good place to meet friends –

Most people can find an exercise class that suits them

and if you join an exercise class with a friend, you are more likely to be disciplined about going each week.

Pilates is a very good alternative to yoga. This is a programme of precise, controlled movements that improve strength and flexibility without bulking up your body. Once the almost-secret province of dancers, Pilates has recently come into its own. Its non-jarring movements and stretches, often machine-assisted, are based on the theory that the abdomen is the body's power centre and that its muscles can anchor strengthening exercises.

If you're more into forced discipline than New Age, you might want to try circuit training. This is an exercise regime that imitates the basic training activities usually reserved for 18-year-old Army recruits. You'll run the obstacle course, hit the ground for push-ups, skip and run sprints before it's all over. It's great for the heart, and it's great for people who like a challenge and not just more of the same. You'll be ready for a good meal after one of these sessions, too!

In other words, exercise, so essential for weight loss and weight control, isn't just dull old calisthenics or 20 minutes on an exercise bike anymore. And the new world of possibilities means there's really no excuse for not exercising.

MONITORING THE MONITOR

If you're accustomed to watching yourself burn calories – literally – on the monitor on your exercise machine, be aware that the reading you get on the monitor is not really accurate. Even if you've entered your age and weight, there are many other variables that affect how many calories you actually burn. The monitor can't give you a precise calorie count.

What the machine monitor can provide, however, is a relative assessment of calorie-burning. In other words, if you continue to use the same machine, you'll be able to compare today's results with the results you get a week or a month from now during the same period of exercise. That way, you can see your improvement over time.

DANCE IT OFF

Want to work your heart, lungs and circulatory system while also learning graceful movement, maintaining low impact and having fun? Try dancing.

Here are just some of the dance exercise programmes available at today's health clubs and leisure centres: Salsa, African dance, Afro-Caribbean dance, Jazz dance, Latin dance, Middle Eastern folk or belly dancing, Reggae and line dancing. All burn calories along with shoe leather, and all are great mood-lifters.

Dance lessons are a good opportunity to meet people, so you won't feel like you're just going for the sake of burning calories. Plus, you'll get inside another culture when you dance to their tune.

ANCIENT MARTIAL ARTS AND MODERN VARIATIONS

Most of the martial arts – developed thousands of years ago in the Orient – evoke images of high-speed punches and whiplash kicks. But that's only part of the picture.

Actually, to perform martial arts correctly, you need training to master the controlled movements. Even Judo, the classic martial art, means 'gentle way'. Despite the grappling and throwing, what judo really teaches is the flexible use of balance, leverage and movement. As an exercise discipline, Judo develops body control, power, flexibility and coordination while also enhancing self-confidence and concentration.

Karate, all the rage among youngsters, offers a great cardiovascular workout while teaching self-defence techniques. It enhances coordination and strength.

In Karate training, students learn to develop a sense of fair play. After every contest, contestants bow to one another in a demonstration of mutual respect.

In Tae Kwon Do, students learn how to use their feet for kick-fighting rather than relying on their hands for defence. The discipline provides an intense strength-building workout that is good for cardiovascular fitness and for flexibility. Like all the martial arts, Tae Kwon Do also helps relieve tension while improving balance and coordination.

Tai chi originated centuries ago in China as a self-defence technique – as well as a religious ritual – but has become the perfect gentle exercise for people of all ages. Part graceful dance-like movements, part slow-motion karate, Tai chi is often called moving meditation. As that phrase implies, it's a great mind-calmer, but it also works the lower body and, of course, the cardiovascular system.

A sequence of Tai chi forms takes your joints through their full range of motion. This martial art also improves coordination and balance, tones muscles, aligns your posture, lowers blood pressure and helps you relax.

In addition to these and other classic martial arts, there are contemporary variations on the theme. Some exercise programmes combine techniques from a range of martial arts disciplines. Others combine martial arts with other aerobic exercises such as dance, running and boxing. Taebo, cardio kickboxing and stepboxkickjump are just some of the names these programmes use. See what your local leisure centre has on offer.

THE SPA EXPERIENCE

Holidays, I think we can all agree, are a time when you should pamper yourself. You want to relax. You want to come back refreshed. You want a break from the everyday whatever-it-is-you-do.

But that doesn't mean a holiday has to be totally sedentary, does it? There are many pleasurable, amusing and leisurely activities to enjoy on your holiday. Far from stressing you out, this is the kind of exercise that can give you a tremendous sense of relaxation and well-being.

If you can afford it, a spa or health-farm break can do wonders for you. It's the kind of break that's offered at many destinations throughout the world. Among these options are day spas, resort spas and destination spas.

A day spa offers beauty, wellness and relaxation programmes on an hourly or daily basis. A resort spa has an 'à la carte' programme that's offered by the resort. A destination spa – the crème de la crème

You can visit a spa for just a few hours or for several weeks

of spa experiences – is devoted exclusively to nutrition, fitness, stress-reduction and wellness. Most destination spas offer an all-inclusive package for several days or weeks.

But why should a spa – any spa – attract you? Firstly, spending time at a spa is a great way to 'get going' on an exercise programme or to take a refresher course if you've allowed yourself to slack off. Secondly, the spa experience provides a wonderful holiday. It includes as much activity as you choose, along with training from experts in case you'd also like that.

Dining policy? Spas specialise in healthy, nutritious meals that taste delicious. If you happen to like cooking, take some classes while you're there, or bring home a catalogue of recipes to make in your own kitchen.

The other plus, of course, is what spas are famous for providing – all the pampering you want. Help yourself to a deep-tissue massage. Have a facial. Or what about a head-to-toe steam cleansing of every pore while you bask in the fragrances offered by aromatherapy?

Spending time at a health farm is also a good way to accustom yourself to incorporating exercise into your lifestyle. Even though the spa experience is truly a holiday – time off from 'real life' – you can still get into the habit of making physical activity an integral part of your existence. In fact, integrating healthy habits into your

FOR THE CALORIE COUNTER

Want to know how many calories you're burning when you rake leaves? How about when you play a set of tennis? While calorie-burning results vary from individual to individual – and depend on a number of factors – the following chart gives at least a relative idea of how effectively you burn calories when you're doing different activities.

Activity	Calories per hour
Cycling	400–700
Running at 6 mph	700
Cross-country skiing	490
Tennis	490
Pushing a lawn mower	420
Swimming	420
Weight training	420
Gardening	350
Low-impact aerobics	350
Walking at 4 mph	315
Raking leaves	280
Tai chi	280
Yoga	280

everyday life is the whole idea behind the spa experience. What differentiates one spa from another is the way the experience is approached, the spa's special style or emphasis.

Given the number of spas today, the variety of their styles, and their geographic range, it's virtually impossible not to find the one that's just right for your own needs. For the weight-conscious, I recommend choosing a spa that emphasises not just the gym workout but outdoor activities as well.

THE 'DO IT' FACTOR

Whatever exercise you choose, whether it's a walk in your local park or a daily session with a personal trainer, the important thing is to just do it. It needn't take a lot of time, and it needn't leave you dripping with sweat and panting for breath. Quite the contrary. Research increasingly demonstrates that

Make exercise an integral part of your everyday lifestyle

brief periods of even low to moderately intense physical activity have benefits for everyone.

It's always possible to find a reason not to exercise. Maybe you love to jog, but not when it's raining. Or the local gym has just upped its fees, and you dropped your membership because you 'don't use it enough'. Or perhaps your enjoyment of long walks takes a nosedive as soon as you have to put on winter clothes.

Exercise, after all, is usually something of an effort. It requires special clothing, or at least a change of clothes. You often need special equipment, such as a racket, knee pads or goggles. Sometimes, you need a team of people. And exercise takes time. If you're

BE HAPPY - EXERCISE

Research studies confirm what people who exercise regularly have long suspected: physical activity can actually make you happier. Some long-term studies suggest that physical fitness and the ability to be active may make people less likely to become depressed. They also even suggest that exercise might be used to treat depression.

Studies have also shown that people who exercise exhibit a more positive outlook on life and are have a greater sense of well-being on a day-to-day basis. It stands to reason: with exercise providing the benefits of weight control, high energy, and feeling good, who wouldn't be happier?

putting in long hours at the office or your home commitments have increased significantly, the days already seem long enough. Fitting exercise into a busy schedule may seem like 'just another thing'.

Remember, though, that exercise is necessary. Do whatever you can to stay motivated. You might have to vary your routines to keep yourself interested. Or you might need to incorporate exercise into your lifestyle, as I suggested earlier, by mowing your own lawn, tending your own garden and so forth.

You might want to try keeping a diary of your workouts: as with your food choices, you will become more aware of what

For weight loss, exercise is a necessity

choices you have made (walking instead of driving, for example). You will also see how closely your workouts and the drop in your waistline are correlated.

THE PSYCHOLOGY FACTOR

WHY DO WE EAT?

Everyone knows the answer to that question: we eat to stay alive, to nourish our bodies, to gain energy and to preserve our health.

We also eat for a range of other reasons. There's the social reason – lunch with a friend, perhaps, or a dinner party. There are also cultural reasons – meals can be the focus of a religious observance, like the Passover Seder, to take one example, or Christmas lunch. We eat to celebrate – what's a birthday cake, after all? – and we even eat when we mourn, such as at a funeral lunch. And, of course, eating plays a role in romance – from the dinner date to breakfast in bed.

But why do some of us overeat? Or eat when we know we're not hungry? Or eat ill-advisedly? Or eat when there's no obvious need or reason at all? The answer to those questions is not so simple. It has to do with emotions, with our own very individual, very personal psychology.

EMOTIONAL EATING

Of course, everyone eats for emotional reasons some of the time. You have an argument with your spouse, and you storm into the kitchen to make a sandwich. Your boss humiliates you, and you take yourself to a lavish lunch – you deserve it after that. You're waiting for your habitually late friend to join you for dinner at the local Indian restaurant, and the minutes drag by like hours, and by the time he arrives, you've eaten a plate of poppadoms and downed two beers. Anger, humiliation, boredom – at the time, each seemed like a good reason for eating, as if food could change your mood.

For some of us, however, the psychology factor influences the totality of our relationships with food. That's why, in my practice, psychology often plays an important role in the weight-loss programme. In fact, whenever a new patient comes through the door, they are seen by three people: a doctor, looking at the problem of being overweight as a total health issue; a nutritionist, who analyses the patient's eating habits and relationship with food; and a psychotherapist, who can help a patient identify the psychological factors that have contributed to the weight problem.

> ### Often, our entire eating pattern is about emotions

Of course, no book can diagnose your particular psychological issues, but knowing how they might be influencing your eating choices is an important component of the awareness that is at the heart of this book. To make thoughtful choices about food, it helps to look not just outwards at the food options you have, but also inwards at the influences that may be compelling you towards one option or another.

In my practice, patients have the option of psychotherapy sessions to help them identify the possible root causes of their eating habits and deal with those causes once and for all, in a supportive, non-judgemental setting. But even if you don't have that option, you can still be aware of the psychological factors that may be influencing your eating habits.

AWARENESS FOR ACTION

Being aware is only the beginning. Once you're aware of an emotional issue affecting your eating habits, you can actually turn that awareness into action to help you control the issue. Every personal insight you glean thus becomes an opportunity for a thoughtful choice. And thoughtful choice is the key to losing weight and keeping it off.

Being aware of internal influences is extremely helpful

For example, food obviously can't resolve a fight with your spouse. Only honest and open communication can do that. What if you simply turned around in the kitchen doorway and went back upstairs to try to work things out? Or at least, what if you took a walk around the block to cool off? Those are two other choices – and for the weight-conscious, better choices.

Nor can food change the humiliation of being yelled at by your boss. Only doing better the next time can fix that problem – or finding a boss who doesn't use humiliation as a management tool. Until either happens, however, why not choose to spend your lunch hour getting rid of your frustrations at the gym?

And certainly, eating a pile of poppadoms and ordering yet another beer will not make your friend arrive any sooner or make the time move any faster. Wouldn't you be better off asking the waiter if there's a spare newspaper around, or using the time to jot down your to-do list for the week? And maybe next time, couldn't you choose to carry a paperback, or adjust the time you tell your friend you'd like to meet, or show up late yourself?

Thoughtful choice, in other words, isn't just about choosing among food options. It's also about being sufficiently in touch with your feelings so that you know why you're making some of the choices you make – and can perhaps step back and choose not to choose.

SEEKING COMFORT, FINDING MORE STRESS

In the cases I've just talked about, the real reason for eating was to find comfort. The angry spouse, the humiliated employee and the bored friend all felt frustrated, upset and stressed out. They wanted to take their minds off what was really happening, and they sought a soothing substitute to do that. What they found was food – familiar, handy, easily available.

For the weight-conscious, however, seeking comfort in eating is like rubbing salt in a wound. You're already angry or stressed or hurt. Eating thoughtlessly only brings you more of what you don't want: added weight and, as a consequence, extra guilt. For you, the

Thoughtless eating will not solve your problems

soothing effect of food is so momentary as to be illusory. It's instant gratification, not lasting satisfaction. Eating will not change the problem that stressed you out in the first place. That problem still exists, but now you've added bad eating choices and the burden of guilt to the problem.

When you're tied up in knots, food won't unravel you. How can it? In fact, if weight loss is your aim, using food as a substitute for comfort often just ties the knots tighter.

FINDING ANOTHER WAY

There are ways to find comfort besides eating high-calorie foods – other activities, other strategies and, always, other foods.

Start by trying to substitute another activity. It should be something other than eating that will provide you with an equivalent gratification while you lower the temperature of your anger or hurt.

I've already mentioned the cooling-off walk around the block, the frustration-busting session at the gym, the paperback or notebook permanently stashed in the

> ## Remember that you always have a choice

handbag or briefcase. Do this kind of comfort-seeking substitute activity often enough, and it will become just as familiar, handy and available as those quick trips to the kitchen, the company cafeteria or the office vending machine.

As another alternative, you could work out a strategy for dealing with the cause of the stress – especially the kind of stress that you know from past experience is likely to send you looking for the bag of crisps or the quick pasta with pesto sauce. Whatever the specifics, make the strategy one that works for your benefit, not against it. Then maybe next time, armed with the strategy, your awareness of the psychology factor at work will empower you to pass up the cheese and onion crisps for the fruit salad – or even for a brisk walk in the park.

From a practical standpoint, having the right foods on hand is a big help. If you're well-stocked with the foods on my Anytime List on page 138, when you storm into the kitchen after an argument with your spouse you'll find food that will give you comfort in a low-calorie way.

As for that friend of yours who's always late: maybe it's time to stop meeting him in restaurants altogether, but if you do, at least it's time to insist that if he's late on this occasion, you're simply going home. Then make sure you stick to your resolve. Your time is too valuable to waste mindlessly scoffing down high-calorie snacks.

STRATEGIC THINKING

Having time on our hands is the classic spur to mindless eating, overeating and high-calorie food choices. As one patient put it, 'When I have nothing to do, I eat to fill the time between meals.'

The same thing goes for the lawyer who retires after 40 years of 12-hour days, only to find himself home, at a loose end, with nothing to do but make trips to the fridge. . . or for the young mother who at last has all three kids in school and finds that time moves at a glacial pace. . . or for the athlete with the broken leg who won't be able to work out again for 3 months.

> ## Finding an alternative strategy can keep you on track

Understanding the cause of the stress lets each of these people create a strategy for dealing with it – and keeps them away from the food cupboards.

What is the cause of their stress? For all three, the thing that gave real meaning and purpose to their lives is gone, and they need to find a replacement, something other than eating that will add to their lives.

Maybe the ex-lawyer can volunteer his time and expertise to a local non-profit organisation that couldn't otherwise afford legal advice. Perhaps the young mother can persuade herself to see her 'empty days' as a blank slate on which she can write a new chapter of her life – maybe by going back to college, volunteering at the hospital or training for a career.

As for the athlete who can't use his legs, he can still use his arms, and he can certainly still use his head. Maybe the local under 12s football team could use another coach, or perhaps it's time to build up those arm, shoulder and pectoral muscles with hand weights.

Finally, let awareness of how your own emotions work become part of your overall thoughtfulness about food. After all, it isn't wrong to eat a bag of crisps or some pasta carbonara, a classically delicious dish, when you're in touch with your feelings about eating it. Simply knowing why you've made a particular choice may lead to another choice next time. As always, I am not telling you not to eat nor asking you to deprive yourself of any food. Quite the contrary. I am asking you to be aware of a range of factors when you make your food choices. One of those factors is psychological.

IS HEALTHY EATING IMPRACTICAL?

Over the years, I've heard almost every conceivable explanation of people's reasons for eating. Unfortunately, some of these explanations are what I would call, simply, excuses. Here are some of the classic excuses for not eating well – and some responses:

Excuse No.1: Health food – even fresh food – is simply too expensive. Eating 'properly' just costs too much.
Response: Actually, it costs less, according to experts at a number of research institutes. An experiment involving people with high blood cholesterol showed that eating heart-healthy food for 9 months cut an average of 70 pence a day off the food bill. For a family of four, that amounts to £1000 a year in financial savings – as well as significant reductions in their cholesterol level and weight, and significant gains in the family's overall health.

Excuse No.2: I don't have the time to eat properly, and I certainly don't have the time to prepare elaborate meals.
Response: Well, how much time do you spend watching television? Hours, probably, and it's safe to say that not all of those hours are illuminating or interesting. What's more, preparing healthy meals need not be inconvenient or time-consuming; see the previous chapter for some shopping tips. Furthermore, eating healthily when you're dining out is possible (*see page 141*).

Excuse No. 3: In my work, I depend on fast food too much to eat properly at lunchtime.
Response: The chances are that your local fast-food place now offers low-calorie, reduced-fat sandwiches and salads. Or try combining a fast-food snack with a more healthy side dish than an order of chips: maybe a salad from the nearby deli's salad bar, or even something brought from home.

PICTURE PERFECT WEIGHT LOSS

PSYCHOLOGY SABOTEURS

There's another way in which the psychology factor may play a role in your weight-loss programme. Just as there are foods that can sabotage your efforts to lose weight and keep it off, there are emotional saboteurs as well. Sometimes the saboteurs are family and friends, but sometimes we do it to ourselves.

A classic example of self-sabotage is the I've-killed-the-day-so-I-might-as-well-really-blow-it syndrome. You're trying to lose weight, and one day at lunch you can't resist temptation, so you eat a piece of chocolate cake. That kills the day.

Since you're having a bad day anyway, you might as well throw caution to the wind and eat that piece of apple pie you think you crave at supper. Since the whole day has then become a failure, you might as well forget the week. After a while, you stop trying to lose any weight at all.

That's a long way to travel from one chocolate dessert. What about just accepting the fact and moving on? You haven't 'killed' anything. You've eaten a delicious dessert. There's nothing bad about it.

Anxiety is natural – but don't let it stop you making choices

Think of trying to push a car up a hill. If it slips a bit, and you catch it and keep pushing, you haven't lost much. If it slips and you let it slide, you'll have to go back down the hill and start all over again. All that earlier effort will have been wasted.

It's the same in weight loss. If you eat the chocolate cake for lunch and keep pushing, you haven't lost much. If you let the chocolate cake kill the day for you, you're back where you started. You then have to

'make up' the entire killed day before you're even at the point where you slipped just a bit. Why climb the same hill twice? Accept the tiny slip, and keep on pushing.

Besides, what's your hurry? This isn't a race. You have undertaken a lifelong commitment to a changed relationship with food. You can afford to lose weight slowly. If things have become uncomfortable for you, wait for a while – even stop until you're comfortable again.

WHEN THE SABOTEUR IS SOMEONE YOU LOVE

It happens more frequently than you think. The husband who has long nagged his wife to lose weight suddenly finds himself living with a glamorous butterfly. She's confronting the world in a whole new way now, and the dynamics of her relationships – with friends, partners and spouse – have changed. You don't have to be a psychologist to know that a change like that can be scary – especially to the husband who lives with the butterfly.

Consciously or unconsciously, he begins acting in ways that actually undermine his wife's weight-loss efforts. He might start bringing home her favourite dessert or insisting on taking her out for lavish restaurant dinners. Maybe he just wants to 'celebrate' her weight loss and doesn't realise that this particular kind of celebrating subverts her success. Most likely, however, he simply doesn't understand the focus of her weight-loss effort. He doesn't understand that she's doing this for herself – for her sense of health and well-being, for her self-esteem, for her own very personal reasons.

She needs to tell him. She must open up those all-important lines of communication and explain exactly why she's doing what she's doing. She needs to assure him that she's not out to attract another man, that he's the one she loves, that she understands his discomfort but that he's reading more into the situation than is there.

Here's a perfect case where the individual can use psychology to overcome psychology, where the wife's awareness of what's going on can empower her to take action that actually helps bring about a new level of closeness in the marriage. When wife and husband communicate clearly, there's a good chance they can work together towards the joint goal of healthy, nutritious, low-calorie eating.

AWARENESS AND ACTION

Have you ever noticed how many extremely accomplished individuals are overweight? I have. My patients include some of the most talented, cultivated, successful people you could ever want to meet. There's no question in my mind that every single one of them – along with every single person reading this book – is capable of losing weight and keeping it off. By understanding the choices available to you, you can be empowered to choose in different ways.

Adding greatly to that understanding is an awareness of the reasons for many of your choices, and of how past choices may have led

Knowing how your own mind works is empowering

to current eating habits. Once you have that awareness, you'll be even better equipped to eat amply, wisely and well for life.

Food, after all, is not the culprit. On the contrary. Food can be – ought to be – a pleasure. The romantic, candlelit dinner. . . the festive Christmas meal. . . the blackberries you and your best friend picked together as kids. . . the haute cuisine banquet in an elegant restaurant. You want to enjoy to the fullest all the reasons for eating that this world has to offer. And you can.

THE PRESSURE TO EAT

In almost all cultures, food has a social significance. It is the centrepiece of family festivities, even of national celebrations. As a result, there is pressure to eat in the way everyone else does. Food can also have personal meaning. For some people, it is their best friend. When they feel alone, food is there to comfort them. As a result, many look forward to being alone with their food at night; it offers the comfort and assurance that they're not getting from other people.

In addition, billions of pounds' worth of advertising urges us to eat at any time of day – all day long. Television, billboards and magazines are constantly pushing mouth-watering images of food. Often, the 'reason' for eating is no reason whatsoever. But advertisers would love us to be constantly thinking about breakfast, snacks, popcorn at the cinema, a hot dog at the football stadium, fast foods, quick lunches, meals in a tin, meals in a snack bar. We can't get away from it. All you can do is be aware of these pressures and think carefully about how they affect you. Don't take orders from a hotdog!

MEETING RESISTANCE AND OVERCOMING IT

Stalled? Well, what happens when you know you're not losing weight anymore? You were going along nicely, shedding pounds at a safe, steady pace. Then nothing. Not last week, the week before last or this week. Something has happened. Your progress has come to a halt. What can you do about it?

The first thing to do is to recognise that a slowdown in the pace of weight loss – even a complete stop – is normal, natural and to be expected. Part of the reason is physical. The fact is, your appetite actually increases after you've undergone weight loss. Picture the fat cells in your body sending SOS messages to your brain – 'Help! We're shrinking! Send fat!' How does the brain respond? By increasing your urge to eat either larger portions or higher-calorie foods. Or both. You answer the urge – often without even being aware that the urge is there – and that, in turn, can slow or stop your weight loss.

> ### Your body fights against any disruption to its equilibrium

But there are other possible reasons for your stall. Maybe there's a subtle, almost imperceptible change in the kinds of foods you're deciding on, or in your eating patterns. Perhaps you're simply bored with the foods you ate with gusto when you started. Or perhaps for some 'very good reason' – there's always a very good reason – you're exercising less than you used to. Maybe a project at work is keeping you in the office from morning till night, too early and too late to get to the gym. Or maybe you usually play tennis, but now winter is setting in and you haven't been able to arrange an indoor court.

At any rate, something may have changed, and the change has slowed or put a halt to your weight loss. In that case you'll need to stand back and re-evaluate the dynamics

> ### You cannot solve a problem until you've analysed it

affecting your weight-control programme. If you think you've gone off track, you need to work out where that happened – and why.

RE-EVALUATING YOUR RELATIONSHIP WITH FOOD

Is something changing your relationship with food? It may be an outside influence, or it may be something from within. To find out what's happening in the case of a stall in weight loss, I've devised a special food diary (see below, opposite). This is a kind of guerrilla tactic to help you find the resistance to your further weight loss and to halt the resistance once you've discovered it. I call it the Direct Action Food Diary.

As with your first food diary (see page 64), you'll note the date and time and provide a description of what you ate, including the amount. Then you'll rate your appetite on a scale of 0 to 4, where 4 is the hungriest. Fill out the first three lines for everything you eat, but for lines four and five, I want you to single out foods you consider either inappropriate or higher in calories than food you would normally allow yourself. For those foods only, write down your mood or feeling before eating and the reason you're eating this food.

After keeping the diary for a week, evaluate what you've written. Focus on the foods you considered inappropriate and turn to the bottom line. Ask yourself this question: if I had it to do all over again, would I eat the higher-calorie food today? In the same circumstances, in the same mood, is there another choice I could have made? What might it be? Write it all down.

The point of using the Direct Action Food Diary is to once again heighten your awareness so that you can determine whether to make changes and what changes you could be making. Remember that the higher-calorie choice is not necessarily an inappropriate one. What counts is the reason for your choice, the thinking behind the decision.

SOME SCENARIOS

Let's say you're having dinner at a friend's home, where the main course is pasta with a carbonara sauce. Usually, you would not choose such a high-calorie pasta dish, but tonight you do – mostly because you're at someone's home, and you don't want to offend your host by rejecting what is served.

The main course is followed by a rich tiramisu for dessert. It looks delicious. As you see it, there's a chance that you have already 'blown' the day with the high-calorie pasta dish, so you decide to eat the tiramisu as well.

When you write up your Direct Action Food Diary that evening, you'll need to fill out the first five lines for both the fettuccine and the tiramisu. Both are higher-calorie dishes than you would normally choose.

When you come to review your choices and fill out line six ('Could I have made another choice?'), the Direct Action Food Diary really shows its worth. As you assess and evaluate the choices you made, it quickly becomes clear that you made one good choice and one not-so-good choice. Given the circumstances, the pasta dish, although high in calories, was a necessary and logical choice. It was the centrepiece of the meal; not eating it would have been truly insulting to your hosts,

who had clearly gone to great trouble to prepare something delicious for you.

Your 'reason' for eating the tiramisu, by contrast, was an excuse. You could easily have said that because the dinner was so good and you ate so much of it, you had no appetite left for the tiramisu, delicious as it looked.

All you had to do was say, 'No, thank you'

Now let's suppose you're at your favourite restaurant one night, and cheesecake is featured on the dessert menu. It's a dessert you love, in a restaurant that is justifiably renowned for its cheesecake and, as it happens, you've eaten low-calorie meals all that day. So you make the choice to order the cheesecake, and you savour every morsel.

Later, as you review your diary and reflect on the choice of cheesecake, you affirm your reasons for making the choice – you wanted it and you had eaten low-calorie foods all day. It was a logical choice, the right choice, not an inappropriate one.

DIRECT ACTION FOOD DIARY

Date/Time _____

Food _____

Hunger level (0–4) _____

Mood/Feeling _____

_____

Why am I eating this now? _____

_____

Could I have made another choice? _____

_____

NEW AWARENESS

Just these few examples are enough to demonstrate why it's so important to keep the Direct Action Food Diary. As you record the simple facts – meal by meal and snack by snack throughout the day – you'll raise your level of awareness and understanding. You really have to stop and think every time you

> **You will find yourself applying fresh thought to your choices**

fill out the food diary. That in itself can be helpful. Many people find that the reason they'd changed their food choices is quite simple – they hadn't been paying attention. What looked like an insurmountable barrier may be out of the way. And your weight loss picks up its pace.

HAS ANYTHING ELSE CHANGED?

There are other possible factors, though. Maybe the change in your eating choices is being propelled by a change in your personal or professional life.

When there's a change for the worse, we find many ways of trying to deal with our misery, depression or sense of loss. Suppose you've ended a relationship or lost a partner, and you're dealing with the unhappiness of being alone, or you're demoted at work and your livelihood is suddenly in jeopardy.

One way to deal with these kinds of stresses is to eat. It's all too simple: there's no need to interact with others; there's no need to think about your actions. All you have to do is open your mouth. What's more, in our society, your misfortune is generally regarded as a reason to eat. You know how it works: a job loss, a death in the family, a spouse's

sickness – if you're battered by such calamities, you owe it to yourself to find comfort in food.

That's all right, so long as you are in touch with the reasons for the changes in your eating. This isn't necessarily a mindless or automatic use of food: it can be deliberate – the giving and receiving of food combines many emotional messages, including sharing, caring and comforting. The point, as always, is to be in touch with the feeling prompting the eating decision.

In fact, any change, good or bad, can produce the kind of stress that makes you think of food. You may be surprised that good changes can create added pressure or stress – but it is so. What if you marry and start a family? Suddenly, you're facing huge new responsibilities. Or you get a splendid promotion at work – and you wonder if you can handle it. These are positive events, and each one carries its payload of stress. One way to deal with that stress is eating.

The bottom line of life changes? It could be the number that shows up on your bathroom scales. When that number stops going down, it's important to review your life, including your relationships, job and

> **At times of stress, we can eat thoughtlessly, without noticing**

living situation, to see what might be causing you the kind of stress that affects your eating habits. It's a good idea to evaluate the ways in which stress-filled events have affected different aspects of your life. Two things in particular may have changed a lot – the amount of exercise you're getting and your degree of motivation. Let's look at those two areas.

EXERCISE

Re-evaluate your commitment to exercise. Has it slipped? Are you exercising less often? Less vigorously? When you go out to exercise, are you spending less time at it?

Even if you are making all the right choices in your eating, a change in the exercise that used to accompany your eating programme can account for the slowdown in your weight loss. You don't need a lot of exercise. But you do need some.

MOTIVATION

You were raring to go when you started, but it's difficult to maintain that level of intensity. The novelty wears off, and instead of attacking each day with charged-up electricity, you feel you're just plodding along. And, as I said earlier in this chapter, the very fact that you've lost weight has actually lowered your need for calories. Technically speaking, to maintain the rate of weight loss you've already experienced, you would have to eat less and less and less. Even then, the weight loss would eventually stop. But of course, we tend to do just the opposite of eating less. All those shrinking cells are yelling 'Feed me!' even louder. Your body wants to eat more – and it wants to eat higher-calorie foods.

A motivational dip, then, is natural. No one can maintain motivation at a high intensity indefinitely. Presumably, once you've identified the change in your eating habits and the cause of the change, once you're again making the kinds of choices that contribute to weight loss, once you again see results, your motivation will also rise. But the fact is that it may not come back to its original energy level. And in a very real sense, isn't that the point? Aren't you trying to make weight control the norm? Don't you want low-calorie choices to be absolutely routine?

Don't despair! The slowed rate of weight loss is no cause for gloom. Don't evaluate your performance by the number on the scales. Think of the weight loss you have achieved, think of how much better you look and feel and applaud yourself.

WHEN GOOD ENOUGH IS GOOD ENOUGH

If what worked before is no longer working, if you've been losing weight steadily and now can't do it, then here's something to consider. Maybe you've gone as far as a weight-loss programme can take you. Maybe wherever you are right now might be the right weight for you. This may be it.

Does that come as good news? Well, not if you secretly long for a certain weight that you think is ideal. Maybe that ideal weight is where you were 5 years ago, or maybe the ideal is being able to fit into a particular dress.

You will have improved your health dramatically

But if this is it, if you've lost all the weight you can reasonably lose – congratulations! You have succeeded in changing your life in enormously positive ways. First of all, if your weight was substantial enough to have put you at risk of heart failure, cancer or diabetes, even a relatively moderate weight loss will have significantly reduced the risk. You will have guaranteed yourself a better quality of life.

You have done wonderful things for your future. Now keep it up – and enjoy the returns the investment yields: increased energy, enhanced self-esteem and an improved appearance. The job of lowering your weight and maintaining good health by changing your relationship with food has been accomplished.

WHAT YOU'LL LOSE, WHAT YOU'LL GAIN

I said at the beginning of this book that weight loss needs to be something that happens while you're still getting on with your life. But it is also true that changing your relationship with food can make your life richer in any number of ways. It isn't just pounds you lose; it's the baggage of being tied to a 'diet', or feeling you must avoid certain situations, or depriving yourself of things you love.

At the age of 26, Mary was one of the shyest people ever to walk through the door of my office. Quiet, modest, diffident, she joined one of the office support groups and almost never said a word. She privately began to see a psychologist about her weight and quietly hired a personal trainer to work with her in her own flat.

What you gain, very often, is the real you

Slowly, as Mary changed more aspects of her relationship with food, more and more weight began to disappear. The exercise began to take effect, toning and sculpting her muscles. The therapy began to take effect, too, as Mary was seen to smile in her support group, then to laugh out loud. And as Mary began to see results, the world began to see the real Mary. This once-shy person began to venture comments that were both funny and insightful. As her appearance changed, she began to get compliments, and soon she was buying a new wardrobe. She took her exercise regime out of the privacy of her home and into the public arena of a gym, where she quickly made friends – even though the sport she took up was boxing! At work, she was promoted to a job of greater responsibility, for more money, with travel to exotic locations.

Today, 2½ stone thinner, Mary finds it easy to be outgoing, to listen to others, to take charge of problems and find solutions. In the same manner, she has taken charge of her food choices and her way of eating.

A NEW LIFE

When Philip first came to see me, he was 76 years old and had just lost his wife to cancer. His suffering took a toll on his body. Philip was chubby round the middle, obviously carrying more weight than was comfortable. His face was pasty-looking, with fleshy jowls, and he moved laboriously, as if weighed down by his sadness. What's more, he had gout, diabetes, heart disease and high cholesterol.

Philip had a simple request to make. 'I've only got 2 more years left,' he told me, 'and I would like to be 2 stone thinner for that time.' So convinced was Philip of the length of time left to him that he initially resisted a physical examination. 'It's not worth it,' he said, 'I'll only be around for 2 more years.'

That was 10 years ago. Today, Philip typically starts his day with a brisk walk – either outdoors or on the treadmill in his flat. Then, as a former businessman, he volunteers his accumulated business wisdom to small start-up companies, and lately he has been perfecting his computer skills. Most evenings are spent out – at a concert or a play, or perhaps having dinner with friends. Of course, Philip lost the 2 stone he wanted to lose – in fact, he lost nearly 4. What he gained, however, was nothing less than a fresh start on a whole new time of life.

THE WEIGHT IS OVER

Of course, I am not promising you that you will add years to your life, or that a funny and fabulous new personality will emerge. What I am promising is that a changed relationship with food will add benefits to your life even as it subtracts pounds and takes away your fear of putting weight back on.

Knowledge is power, as the saying goes, and the knowledge you gain from this book can give you the power you need to change your relationship with food. First of all, you should now have a realistic sense of just what is an appropriate goal for you. Genetic predisposition and even psychological factors can affect your weight. Therefore, for the person you are, there's an appropriate weight at which you'll look and feel your best. That's the goal you want to aim for and maintain.

Secondly, the nutritional knowledge you glean from this book provides the essential tools you'll need to get to that goal and stay there. I'm sure that the visual demonstrations are burned into your brain. Now, more often than not, when you see one kind of food that you might have eaten impulsively, you also see vivid images of the other lower-calorie choices.

LOOKING BEYOND

Gaining an understanding of how to read nutrition labels and learning to look behind the 'low-fat' or 'low-sugar' labels to the calorie numbers are equally important. So is an awareness of the wide range of foods that you may have been surprised to find are not at all 'forbidden'.

Further, what you've learned in these pages doesn't end when you close the book. You now have a basis on which you can build. As new studies provide new information on nutrition, you're equipped to assess what they mean. As new food products come on the market, you know enough to be able to determine if they should be added to your own personal list of options.

> **If the images start to fade, the pictures are always here**

What's more, when you have undertaken the programme in this book, you have the power forever. Once you have gone through Food Awareness Training and have become a mindful eater in the driver's seat of your food choices, you possess all the tools you'll ever need to maintain an appropriate weight for the rest of your life.

GAINING BY LOSING

I promise you that a changed relationship with food – combined with regular physical activity – will make you a healthier person. What's more, the soundness and fitness that come from healthy eating and regular exercise invariably coincide with a more cheerful and positive attitude, with a higher energy level, and even with clearer thinking and a stronger sense of well-being. For the rest of your life, the quality of your life will be better. It's a lot to gain.

And you don't have to go hungry, look or act like you're 'on a diet', give up your favourite foods, abstain from alcohol, join a gym or be afraid you'll gain back the weight you shed. Isn't it time you started changing your relationship with food? After all, what have you got to lose?

CONVERSION CHARTS

These equivalents have been slightly rounded to make measuring easier.

VOLUME MEASUREMENTS

METRIC	IMPERIAL
5ml	1 tsp
15ml	1 tbsp
30ml	1 fl oz
60ml	2 fl oz
80ml	3 fl oz
120ml	4 fl oz
150ml	5 fl oz ($^1/_4$ pint)
180ml	6 fl oz
200ml	7 fl oz ($^1/_3$ pint)
240ml	8 fl oz
300ml	10 fl oz ($^1/_2$ pint)
350ml	12 fl oz
400ml	14 fl oz
500ml	18 fl oz
600ml	20 fl oz (1 pint)

CALORIES TO KILOJOULES (kJ)

Calories x 4.186 = Kilojoules

CALORIES	KILOJOULES (kJ)
1	4.186
10	41.86
25	104.65
50	209.3
75	313.95
100	418.6
200	837.2
300	1255.8
400	1674.4
500	2093
600	2511.6
700	2930.2
800	3348.8
900	3767.4
1000	4186

WEIGHT MEASUREMENTS

METRIC	IMPERIAL
15g	$^1/_2$ oz
30g	1 oz
50g	$1^3/_4$ oz
60g	2 oz
75g	$2^1/_2$ oz
100g	$3^1/_2$ oz
115g	4 oz ($^1/_4$ lb)
125g	$4^1/_2$ oz
145g	5 oz ($^1/_3$ lb)
170g	6 oz
200g	7 oz
230g	8 oz ($^1/_2$ lb)
285g	10 oz
340g	12 oz ($^3/_4$ lb)
400g	14 oz
455g	16 oz (1lb)
500g/$^1/_2$ kg	1lb 2 oz
600g	1lb 5 oz
1kg	2.2lb

LENGTH MEASUREMENTS

METRIC	IMPERIAL
0.6cm	$^1/_4$ inch
1.25cm	$^1/_2$ inch
2.5cm	1 inch
5cm	2 inches
11cm	4 inches
15cm	6 inches
20cm	8 inches
25cm	10 inches
30cm	12 inches (1ft)

INDEX

Boldface page references indicate boxed text and tables.
Italic references indicate photographs.

ACKNOWLEDGMENTS

173

ACKNOWLEDGMENTS

In writing this book I have learned that authorship is a lot like medicine: both are collaborative processes. I'm glad for this opportunity to acknowledge and thank the many people who helped make *Dr Shapiro's Picture Perfect Weight Loss* a reality.

First and unquestionably foremost, I owe a debt of gratitude to nutritionist Phyllis Roxland. A friend and colleague of 20 years' standing, Phyllis was not only instrumental in formulating the principles of the weight-loss programme, she also helped with every aspect of this book, often putting her personal life on hold to do so. I am thankful not only for the weekends sacrificed but also for the dedication that kept me focused on the task at hand. This book simply would not have been possible without Phyllis Roxland.

In helping to shape and polish the original US version of this book, writer Susanna Margolis and Ed Claflin, my editor at Rodale, offered intelligence and much-appreciated humour along with considerable professional expertise. They helped me express my thoughts – sometimes, it seemed, before they were even formulated in my mind – and they were a pleasure to work with. Kay von Bergen's creativity spurred my own and gave birth to the book's title, while her generous spirit sustained and supported the overall effort. My thanks also to Abbie Claflin whose involvement in the book's creation was brief but memorable.

Mel Berger, my agent at the William Morris Agency, grasped the concept of the book at the early stages and staunchly advocated the use of colour photography, an element I believe is essential to the book's message.

Diane Vezza, ably assisted by Joan Parkin and Rose Holden, brilliantly styled the subjects of the photography in the original US edition, which were beautifully brought to life by photographer Kurt Wilson and his assistant Troy Schnyder – all under the superb direction of James Gallucci, Rodale's photo editor. Thanks go to photographer Jeremy Hopley and photography assistant Clare Miller for their work on this new edition.

In designing the original US edition, senior book designer Christina Gaugler exhibited not just great talent but superb organisational savvy as well. I would like to thank Sharon Rudd, Amanda Lunn, Laura Watson and Briony Chappell for their help on the redesign and production of this new edition.

A special thanks to Anne-Laure Lyon, friend and fashion stylist, whose keen eye and sense of style made such a difference.

I felt warmly welcomed, encouraged and supported by Rodale's incomparable publishing professionals in producing this new edition of the book. On the editorial and production front, I am grateful to Maggie Ramsay, Laura Seber, Kate Hayward, Jane Baldock, Margaret Cornell, Aaron Brown, Elizabeth Mallard-Shaw, Anne Lawrance, Keith Bambury and Sara Granger for all their effort. Special thanks to home economist Annie Nichols and dietician Sue Baic. And I am also pleased to acknowledge those at Rodale who helped make this book a reality: Tami Booth, Adrian Webster and Sean Moore.

I am particularly grateful to Cindy Ratzlaff for the great confidence she showed in planning and implementing publicity for the US version of this book. Cindy was ably assisted by a superb trade-book marketing and promotion team that includes Renee James, Shannon Gallagher and Mary Lengle. The publicity campaign certainly contributed to the overwhelming success of the US version, and that, in turn, has prompted this new edition. The staff in my New York office deserves – and gets – my deepest thanks. On a daily basis they dealt with my sometimes frantic effort to be both physician and author. They consistently exhibited equanimity of spirit while supporting the effort in very practical terms. I extend my most heartfelt gratitude to office staffers Gerri Pietrangolare, Alexandra Lotito, Shanette Vega and Catherine Fallon; to nutritionist Marcia Cohen; to psychologists Dr Stephanie Secolsky, Dr Norman Wyloge and Linda Charnes, MFT; and to physical therapist Yuri Usher. A special thank you to Susan Amato, CSW, for her contributions to the chapters on the psychology of weight loss, and for her ongoing support of this project and her enthusiastic participation.

Support and enthusiasm were also offered in great measure by my brother, Michael Shapiro, and my sister, Marilyn McLaughlin. I'm grateful to them both. Thanks also to my dogs, Willow and Barkley, for uncharacteristically failing to eat the manuscript of the book.

Finally, I want to thank my patients – all those I have worked with over the past 25 years. You have been the proving ground for the principles of *Dr Shapiro's Picture Perfect Weight Loss* programme, and your enthusiasm, dedication and commitment to those principles – as well as the successes you've achieved – have quite simply been my inspiration.

Dr Howard M. Shapiro

OTHER RODALE BOOKS
AVAILABLE FROM PAN MACMILLAN

1-4050-0666-8	Banish Your Belly, Butt & Thighs Forever!	*The Editors of* Prevention *Health Books for Women*	£10.99
1-4050-4099-8	Before the Heart Attacks	*Dr H Robert Superko*	£10.99
1-4050-4179-X	Fit not Fat at 40+	Prevention *Health Books*	£12.99
1-4050-0665-X	Get A Real Food Life	*Janine Whiteson*	£12.99
1-4050-0667-6	The Green Pharmacy	*Dr James A. Duke*	£14.99
1-4050-0673-0	The Home Workout Bible	*Lou Schuler*	£15.99
1-4050-2101-2	8 Minutes in the Morning	*Jorge Cruise*	£12.99
1-4050-0672-2	Pilates for Every Body	*Denise Austin*	£12.99
1-4050-3338-X	The *Runner's World* Complete Book of Running	*Amby Burfoot*	£18.99
1-4050-0669-2	The Testosterone Advantage Plan	*Lou Schuler*	£11.99

All Pan Macmillan titles can be ordered from our website, *www.panmacmillan.com,* or from your local bookshop and are also available by post from:

Bookpost, PO Box 29, Douglas, Isle of Man IM99 1BQ
Credit cards accepted. For details:
Telephone: 01624 836000
Fax: 01624 670923
E-mail: bookshop@enterprise.net
www.bookpost.co.uk

Free postage and packing in the United Kingdom.

Prices shown above were correct at time of going to press.

Pan Macmillan reserve the right to show new retail prices on covers which may differ from those previously advertised in the text or elsewhere.

For information about buying *Rodale* titles in **Australia**, contact Pan Macmillan Australia. Tel: 1300 135 113; fax: 1300 135 103; e-mail: *customer.service@macmillan.com.au*; or visit: *www.panmacmillan.com.au*

For information about buying *Rodale* titles in **New Zealand**, contact Macmillan Publishers New Zealand Limited. Tel: (09) 414 0356; fax: (09) 414 0352; e-mail: *lyn@macmillan.co.nz*; or visit *www.macmillan.co.nz*

RODALE

MACMILLAN